A Life in Medicine

A British Doctor's Account

A Life in Medicine

A British Doctor's Account

G. C. Cook, MD, DSc, FRCP, FRCPE, FRACP, FLS
Visiting Professor, University College London

TROPZAM

Copyright © G C Cook 2024
First published in 2024 by TROPZAM
11 Old London Road, St Albans, Herts, AL1 1QE

Distributed by Gardners Books, 1 Whittle Drive, Eastbourne, East Sussex, BN23 6QH
Tel: +44(0)1323 521555 | Fax: +44(0)1323 521666

www.amolibros.com
Cover image: One of the last cases of smallpox in southern Nigeria, photographed by the author in 1961.

The right of G C Cook to be identified as the author of the work has been asserted herein in accordance with the Copyright, Designs and Patents Act 1988.

All rights reserved. This book is sold subject to the condition that it shall not, by way of trade or otherwise, be lent, resold, hired out or otherwise circulated without the publisher's prior consent in any form of binding or cover other than that in which it is published and without a similar condition including this condition being imposed on the subsequent purchaser.

British Library Cataloguing in Publication Data
A catalogue record for this book is available from the British Library.

ISBN 978-0-9560598-6-4

Typeset by Amolibros, Milverton, Somerset
This book production has been managed by Amolibros
Printed and bound by T J Books Ltd, Padstow, Cornwall, UK

The London *Times* newspaper began new year 2023 with a bold heading:

A&E [now a National Health issue (and previously the 'envy of the world') delays are] killing up to 500 patients every week.

and later that year:

A&E delays put patients in danger … fears raised as total NHS waiting list hits 7.7. m[illion].

and later still:

Uncaring profession: for the first time, NHS consultants and junior doctors will this week strike on the same day. This reckless escalation makes them unworthy of public respect.*

---

* R Blakeley, H Zeffman. A&E delays 'killing up to 500 patients every week: senior medics warning as hospitals struggle with staff shortages, surgery backlogs, flu and Covid. *Times*, Lond 2023 2 January: 1; K May. A&E delays put patients in danger, says doctor: fears raised as total NHS waiting list hits 7.7m. *Ibid* 15 September: 1, 2: Anonymous. Uncaring profession: For the first time, NHS consultants and junior doctors will this week strike on the same day. This reckless escalation makes them unworthy of public respect. *Ibid* 18 September.

CONTENTS

List of Illustrations	viii
Preface	1
Prologue	5
1 Before the *National Health Service* (NHS)	8
2 Medical training: I. pre-clinical	12
3 Medical Training: II. Clinical	19
4 The pre-registration years	23
5 *After National Service* – 1962 onwards	27
Epilogue	41
APPENDIX: Nutritional research in southern Africa:	53
My *'academic'* contributions in Zambia	53
Index	77

List of Illustrations

Fig 1: Group of newly qualified junior doctors in 2023 – on strike for an increase in pay. P Brookes. ***Times, Lond* 2023; 21 September: 25**   21

Fig 2: Letter from the foremost expert on fructose metabolism (Professor H A Krebs FRS) during my research spell on sucrose at the Department of Medicine, the *Royal Free Hospital School of Medicine.*   30

Fig. 3: Telegram offering the Chair of Medicine in the University of Zambia to the author.   32

Fig 4: Letter from Lord Rosenheim FRCP, FRS to Lusaka in which he expressed his great pleasure at being invited to be external examiner in the first final examination in Medicine at the *University of Zambia.*   33

Fig 5: Britain was at that time afflicted by numerous strikes for an increase in pay with widespread implications. P Brookes.
***Times, Lond* 2023: 2 September: 23.**   40

Preface

In July 2022, the London *Sunday Times* had used as its front-page headline:

It's no longer feasible to be a *full-time GP* [general practitioner]: doctors' leader warns of working hours crisis.[1]

I well recall the days when healthcare in Britain was very different from that of today. There was no *health service* and the era of antibiotics had not yet arrived. These were days with which the younger generation of today is obviously *not* familiar. How could they be? The antibiotic age only began in the 1940s, and the *National Health Service* (NHS) came into operation in 1948, the Act having been passed two years earlier. Health and prevention of disease as we presently know them in Britain thus began in 1948 which only very old folk, such as myself, can remember.

The political promise, in 1948, of *free* healthcare for *all* from 'cradle to grave' sounded of course simply 'too good to be true' while in 2024 (after 75 years) it seemed totally senseless! Had more time been spent in the years following WWII (1939-45) in *creation* of the NHS we might not be where we are now, for since the time of the monasteries or before it had been the *poor* who were targeted for healthcare, and not the rich who could always afford to pay for it themselves but merely used it for financial gain; the wealthy have thus exploited the NHS! Also, *preventive* strategies should have been incorporated at its outset. In many respects of course, the scheme was totally laudable! It is therefore of little surprise that younger generations are *only* aware of the NHS and antibiotic eras, and nothing before.

While trained at considerable expense by the British government *via* a *Surrey Country Council Scholarship* to work in this country, I make *no* apology for spending much of my medical career in the 'third world'. Now that Britain is totally corrupt from a former Prime Minister downwards[2], together with rapidly declining religious belief in the *West*[3], assistance to *developing countries* seemed right!

It is likely too that the antibiotic era will historically be only a transitory period in human history; events of the 1940s and beyond will loom large in the future. The antibiotic age will terminate sometime in the relatively near future as Alexander Fleming (1881-1955) suggested it would [4], and requests for penicillin or one of its successors from the general practitioner will inevitably end. In the words of one recent British Prime Minister (certainly not Boris Johnson), from a health angle the present population of Britain 'has never had it so good'.

Accreditation of the true place of antibiotics in the *twenty-first* century is to some extent controversial; the present younger generation has in fact grown up in a curious and unprecedented (*antibiotic*) era. When I was a child they simply did *not* exist and we could *not* therefore run to our GP for a course every time we had a cough or cold! Antibiotics then, only date from the 1940s in a world which is millions of years old, and Fleming (*see above*) himself realised that bacterial *resistance* was merely on the horizon (*see above*). Therefore, between the 1940s and today *Homo sapiens* has lived in effect in a totally 'false' environment; following its multi-million-year history, mankind has thus been living for some 70 to 80 years in a man-made scenario, and most certainly not one which has existed forever! While they remain effective they should be reserved for a proven infection.[5]

Just as later in this book when great controversy erupted regarding the state of the nationalised practice of medicine, the air in the 1950s and 60s had remained full of the contentious matter of the desirability of female doctors despite the pioneering work of the *London School of Medicine for Women*. In 1922 the London *Times* newspaper had even spoken of a 'ban on *new* women medical students' at the London Hospital, whilst there were [at that time] *no* women at Guy's. It seems that male sports (headed by rugby football) had an important part to play.[6]

What is the child with a gift for learning to do in 2024? He/she is not now in a world of learning moulded by centuries of scholarship, but by one of materialism inspired by Margaret Thatcher.[7]

I was born in 1932 and there's no way I would read medicine today. Gone are the days of the *great profession*, the discipline having been taken over by vote-gathering politicians who have in most cases received *no* training in medicine while I would have become a mere *civil servant*. During my lifetime therefore, I have witnessed both initiation of healthcare by politicians and the end of the 'reign' of the properly trained medical profession. In the meantime, the *free National Health Service* (NHS) became 'the envy of the world'. This book describes my personal experiences during those years and their sad departure.[8]

Maureen Moran has kindly typed the book from my longhand.

References and notes

1. T Calver. 'It's no longer feasible to be a full-time GP': doctors' leader warns of working hours crisis. *Sunday Times, Lond* 2022; 24 July: 1; K Lay, M Hendrix, R Watts. GPs long hours are anti-women and should be cut, say doctors. *Times, Lond* 2022; 25 November: 13.
2. C Midgley. Cheers, Boris, I'm going to follow your lead and turn to a life of crime. *Times 2, Lond* 2022; 25 May: 2.
3. K Burgess. Religious 'contagion' rate reveals dying churches. *Times, Lond* 2022; 25 May: 20; A Vaughan. Antibiotic-resistant bugs found in rivers. *Ibid* 2022; 22 November: 1415; P B Baker. Antibiotics hazard. *Ibid*; 25 November:32; D White. Antibiotics may be given en masse in schools after Strep A kills nine. *Ibid* 2022; 7 December: 8; K Burgess. End of an era for Christian Britain. *Ibid* 2022; 30 November: 7; D Aaronovitch. As an atheist, declining religion worries me: our places of worship help to bind communities and we should focus on their role even as active faith is on the wane. *Ibid* ; 1 December: 27; Correspondence: Decline of religious observance in Britain. *Ibid:* 1 December: 30; Correspondence. Value of religion or community glue. *Ibid*; 2 December: 36; M Syed. We're losing our religion, what will fill the void? 'More than a third of our population now do not belong to any faith. Turning away from gods may be inevitable, but we risk losing a powerful source of comfort. *Sunday Times, Lond* 2022; 4 December: 30.
4. P Watkins. *From Hell Island to Hay Fever: the life of Dr Bill Frankland*. Bath, England 2018: 282; Correspondence column. Reducing the prescription of a pill for each ill. *Times, Lond* 2022; 20 June: 28;
5. K Lay. Steep growth in infections that defy antibiotics a 'serious threat'. *Ibid* 2020; 19 September: 22.
6. Anonymous. More views on women doctors [in 1922]. *Ibid* 2022; 4 March: 34; Anonymous. Challenges to women in medicine [in 1923]. *Ibid* 2023; 2 October: 26.
7. T Owalade. Nurtured, a love of learning is a lifelong gift; childlike curiosity can be dulled by our exposure in waves of 'junk food' that is easily consumed but has little real value. *Times, Lond* 2023; 2 January: 21.
8. P Morland. *A Fortunate Woman: a country doctor's story*. London: Picador 2022: 236.

Prologue

Although this book is centred on my personal experience(s) within healthcare in Britain and 'developing' countries in the last century, it also contains reflections on widespread disquiet with its availability in the last few decades – principally resulting from transfer from a mature medical profession to 'amateur' governance by untrained politicians. The state of healthcare in Britain has rightly come in for a great deal of criticism; can it all be a result of the recent Covid-19 pandemic? After all, the Tory party, for a time under the renowned liar Boris Johnson, held the office of Prime Minister for a decade and more!

The national healthcare system has for over the last half-century been in the hands of politicians, having wrestled it from its rightful 'owner', *ie* the *medical profession*. Several articles in a leading newspaper succinctly summarised the current situation in banner headlines on its front page:

'Majority now expect delays in NHS treatment'

- Almost half think [the] service is getting worse,
- Six in 10 appointment waits [are] unreasonable.[1]

A ¾ page article is entitled:

- Will we ever trust our politicians again?[2]

And the entire leading article is titled:

- When voters lose faith in the NHS, Westminster must listen.[3]

When in 1948 the NHS was introduced, it should have been targeted at the 'poor off'. Instead, the 'well-off' were included and the '*free*' service for *all* became virtually impossible on financial grounds.

This was of course a most interesting time in which to study medicine; in 1948 the *National Health Service* came into operation promising healthcare from 'cradle to grave'. The NHS functioned well at first and then ran out of money. To my mind those who developed this new way of administering healthcare in the UK made a serious error in including all and sundry in this *free* service. That the poor were 'catered' for was highly praiseworthy but to include the rich (who could well afford healthcare) was unnecessary and led to the future downfall of a highly desirable scheme.

By 2023 there was a great tendency to blame every fault on the recent Covid-19 pandemic, instead of acknowledging that far more should have been done *before* the present situation arose!

Thus, since introduction of the NHS in 1948, the political party in power has theoretically been responsible for the NHS and that party has gained as much credit as possible for its *free* service but kept relatively quiet when adverse effects arose.

When the British government acquired healthcare in the name of the NHS they took over many hospitals from previous decades and even centuries, a few of which they subsequently re-built. The very long history of care of the poor can be traced in books dating from Britain's medieval years; in retrospect it has become abundantly clear that it is the poorer classes who should have been targeted in some way on the structure of the nascent NHS. The 'rich' have always been able to afford healthcare. By 2024, the NHS had become moribund and the $64,000 question was with what to replace it. It had been the 'envy of the world' and admired by many. But it was costing too far much to run! Its future is beyond the scope of this book.[4]

References

1. S Lintern, G Wheeler. Majority now expect delays in NHS treatment. *Sunday Times, Lond* 2022; 28 August: 1; E Yeomans. Student died from sepsis after suspected spider bite *Times, Lond* 2022; 3 December: 21.
2. T Calver. Will we ever trust our politicians again? *Ibid:* 17.
3. Anonymous (leading article). When voters lose faith in the NHS, Westminster must listen. *Ibid:* 20.
4. C Renwick. *Bread For All: the origins of the welfare state.* London; Allen Lane 2017: 323; G Barry, L A Carruthers. *A history of Britain's hospitals: and the background to the medical, nursing and allied professions.* Sussex, England; Book Guild Publishing 2005: 430; L Granshaw, R Porter (eds). *The Hospital in History.* London; Routledge, Chapman and Hall 1989: 273; E M McInnes. *St Thomas' Hospital.* London; Special Trustees for St Thomas' Hospital, London 1963: 288; R Colville. Politicians used to have a vision to save the NHS. You won't hear them being so bold today: its values are right, but its structures are wrong. It still has the feel of the 1940s. *Sunday Times, Lond* 2022; 11 December: 28.

Chapter One

Before the National Health Service (NHS)

I can well recall events *before* creation of the *National Health Service* (NHS) when Medicine was still a highly respected profession, often bracketed with Law and the (Anglican) church; this was in some ways a relic of the Victorian age. An overview of the profession in Britain from early times is provided by Mervyn Herbert shortly before World War II, with particular attention to its administration. There is also coverage of the forthcoming *nationalised* organisation (the NHS), this transition being shortly after my own medical career began. Now, as many as one in every seven citizens of the UK is denied a general practitioner (GP)'s appointment! I am thus relatively unusual in that I have experienced the entire span of the NHS.[1]

Before introduction of the NHS in 1948 we were forced to use medicaments including herbal remedies which had been used by our 'grandmothers' and past generations, instead of antibiotics (prescribed under the NHS) for any manner of cough and cold. I was reminded of this when the first page of the London *Times* reminded its reader(s) that honey (rather than antibiotics) for coughs and colds was effective.[2] Those of us who were brought up with Victorian remedies to the fore, are less likely to rush to his/her GP for an antibiotic for a trivial infection which in any case is unlikely to respond to an antibiotic! A cough/cold only occasionally demands an urgent request for an antibiotic – assuming the cause is a virus it will *not* respond to an antibiotic anyway!

As a child of the 1930s, I vividly recall visits from the family's general practitioner who lived and practised several roads from ours in Wimbledon Park, South-west London; his name was Carter and I am sure he trained in Edinburgh – still a stronghold of British medicine. Each time I or my brother or sister developed one of the childhood infections, Dr Carter was soon in attendance. A later GP was Dr Clunies-Ross – one of the family of that name living in the Cocos Islands.[3] My father could recall the days when GPs arrived well-dressed and wearing a top hat, etc.

We children all received appropriate 'vaccines' for childhood diseases which were accepted without question; the 'anti-vax movement' remained in the distant future. Although infective disease was then a common entity, most people believed in the *excellent* beneficial results of immunisation (or vaccination for smallpox). I remember being immunised at my school, the Wimbledon Park Primary School – thank goodness I was never to enter a *public* school – in 1937 and being roundly scolded by my mother, because my father considered *private* immunisation to be superior! Then there was *cod liver oil and malt* which recent work has confirmed to be effective in management of tuberculosis.

After one of Carter's visits, I recall asking my mother what was meant by 'having one's bowels open'; this was followed by a somewhat and mildly embarrassed silence.

Infectious disease was so prevalent that talk of yet another child in the same road as ours being smitten with *scarlet fever, poliomyelitis, pneumonia* or perhaps *appendicitis* was by no means unusual. I recall too a neighbour who died of Paget's Disease of Bone – now a disease of the past. Mongolism (Down's Syndrome) also seemed common in that suburb.

Following my childhood experiences, there is a void in my memory until my teenage years were virtually over!

Until then it was generally considered that the ancient Greeks were pioneers in elucidation of the anatomy of the body of *Homo sapiens*, which in those days we had to dissect as medical students (*see below*). However, relatively recent research suggests that the Chinese were the first to reveal *Homo sapiens*' anatomy; this was revealed working through ancient *silk* manuscripts at least 800 years old discovered in the 1970s, and anatomical texts, while in the West dissection of the *human* body was 'frowned upon'; the authors then would only have had access to bodies of criminals.[4]

Medicine as a career?

My school history is briefly outlined in an autobiography written in 2011.[5] I was intent on pursuing a career in Zoology. When I was approaching the end of my school career, I had a talk with my Biology 'master' – Dr Tom Bamford PhD – at Raynes Park Grammar School, who advised me that a career in Medicine (which then remained a highly ranked profession) was not outside my capability. Pursuance of this highly prestigious profession immediately appealed to me, especially as it was geared to benefits to 'humanity' unlike Zoology; thus I was to cease dissecting earthworms, dogfish and rabbits and soon revert to *H sapiens*. In the 1950s, a career in medicine tended to be more altruistic than today, and not oriented on making a fortune; strikes were simply unknown. This change of tack did not go down well with my mother – who immediately opposed my change from Zoology. My father had little to say, but certainly did *not* in any way attempt to change my mind.

Differing face of Medicine

A major difference in 2024 in my view therefore is that Britain has become far more *materialistic,* primary concern now being financial. I joined this *great profession* not to become a civil servant and to gain financially. This has been admirably confirmed by an immigrant Muslim (known to me) and now in a senior medical position who seems to have developed an obsessive love of cash.

Although medical 'progress' during my lifetime has rightly decreased human mortality in developing countries, world over-population has inevitably resulted. A most unnatural event is happening in Britain – mean age of women when giving birth has risen, according to the *Office for National Statistics,* to 30.7 years. This departure from the natural scheme of things is resulting in another change from normality involving women; there is a movement to *encourage* larger families again. We all know about China but now a relatively new leader in Japan has stressed that as his first priority, he wants *more* babies to be born. This new 71-year-old Prime Minister– Yoshihide Suga (1948-present) – faces the post-world war II 'baby boom' when the country was 'flooded' with children who have now 'disappeared'! The *elderly* are now about to make up one-third of the population. But this is not a recent matter and various solutions have been suggested:

- make motherhood more attractive; better creches and nursery care, etc, and

- introduction of a 'home town tax'; people in cities can choose to pay council tax to a *rural* government other than the one in which they live.

But today, Japanese simply don't want large families – a situation which is expected to last.[6]

References and notes

1. S M Herbert. *Britain's Health* London: Penguin Books, Ltd 1937:219; K Lay, C Smyth. 1 in 7 denied GP appointment: millions of patients turned away – while others wait for over a month – as Labour vows to train more doctors. *Times, Lond* 2022; 6 December 1.
2. K Lay. If you need to beat a cough, honey takes the biscuit. *Ibid* 2020; 19 August: 1; K Southern. Honey, we're home: 6,000 bees move in. *Ibid* 2022; 22 June: 32; R Campbell-Johnson. Anatomy laid bare: the ghoulish art of medical and scientific adventure. *Ibid* 2022; 25 June: *Saturday Review:* 8-9; G C Cook. *Before the 'Germ Theory': a history of cause and management of infectious disease before 1900*. Ely, Cambridgeshire; Melrose Books 2015: 202; J Blackburn. Baked owl, roasted puppy prescriptions, medieval style. *Times, Lond* 2022; 18 August: 201-1; R Blakely. Vinegar and honey on prescription? *Ibid* 2023; 13 July: 14. (*See also*: J Wesley. *Primitive Physick; or, an easy and natural method of curing most diseases.* Bristol: William Fine 1770: 156.)
3. The Clunies-Ross family were the original settlers in the Cocos (Keeling) Islands, a small archipelago in the Indian Ocean. From 1827 to 1978, the family ruled the previously uninhabited islands as a private fiefdom, initially as *terra nullius* and later under British 1857-1955) and Australian (1955-1978) sovereignty. The head of the family was usually recognised as the resident magistrate, and was sometimes styled as "King of the Cocos Islands", a title given by the press.
4. G Wilford. Ancient scripts show Chinese studied anatomy before Greeks. *Times Lond* 2020 3 September: 3.
5. G C Cook. *Torrid Disease: memoirs of a tropical physician in the late twentieth century.* St Albans: Amolibros 2011: 277.
6. Anonymous. New high as average age for giving birth rises to near 31. *Times, Lond* 2020; 17 November: 14; R L Parry. New leader, 71, must persuade Japanese to have more babies. *Ibid* 2020; 19 September: 45.

Chapter Two

Medical training: I. pre-clinical

Of course, having decided on a medical career, I still had to obtain a place at a Medical School. I was interviewed at numerous London medical schools without success. I recall Bart's, Guy's, Middlesex, and Charing Cross (there might have been others also) and finally the *Royal Free*. Nowadays only 40% of doctors are apparently UK-trained. Furthermore, owing to increased interference from UK Government it is difficult for a UK national (rather than a 'foreign' individual) to obtain a place in a UK-based medical school.[1]

In those distant days it was usual for the eldest son to attend a public school and then take over the GP practice from his father. I did not possess this family tradition so was thus delighted to be offered a place at this poorly ranked 'citadel' of women's medicine situated at Euston, London.

The **Royal Free Hospital** had been founded by William Marsden (1796-1867) in 1828 to provide *free* healthcare to those who could not otherwise afford medical treatment. The Royal Charter had been granted by Queen Victoria (1819-1901) in 1837, recognising work on *cholera* (*see below*)[2] during the *nineteenth* century. For many years, the 'Free' had been the only London hospital to offer medical training for women – later becoming the *Royal Free Hospital School of Medicine*. In the 1970s the hospital moved to Hampstead from its previous 'home' in Gray's Inn Road – amalgamating the parent hospital with its various branches – at Lawn Road, Liverpool Road, New End and Hampstead General (all later subsumed by the NHS).[3]

While I was an undergraduate, the ancient Greek physician *Hippocrates* was frequently referred to as the 'rôle model' for all recruits to the *profession*, and in addition to his enunciation of ethical principles in the practice of medicine, he probably also contributed much more than formerly recognised regarding

Greek literature. Now that medical practice merely consists of the life of a civil servant, that immediately assumes less importance and those basic ethical tenets have become virtually extinct. In a recent study methodological texts involving patients' symptoms in which he gave detailed case-histories, etc, are thought to date to about 410 BC, although earliest ones were probably written in around 470 BC – he certainly does *not ascribe illness 'to the gods'*. It is likely also that *epidemics* influenced Thucydides, an historian (father of *scientific* history). Recently researched texts set him apart from contemporary medicine in Egypt, Babylon and numerous other societies.

The '*Royal Free*' (RFH – *see also* above) has a highly distinguished history, first seeing the 'light of day' in Hatton Garden, London in 1828, where its founder Marsden (*see above*), had witnessed a young woman die, probably from *tuberculosis* (but syphilis has not been excluded), which was rife in early *nineteenth* century London, as an entirely altruistic exercise. After a series of negotiations with the *London School of Medicine for Women* (later the RFHSM) formed the first venue for female education in medicine worldwide, as a *teaching* hospital. Of course the London medical scene had been dominated by teaching foundations very much older than this one – beginning with the ancient St Bartholomew's founded by a monk as long ago as AD 1123. Also Thomas Linacre (1460-1524) founded the (Royal) College of Physicians in 1518.

It is perhaps somewhat insulting to find a description of the *Royal Free* as 'one of the least regarded medical schools in London' in an otherwise excellent account of the 'Andrew Wakefield saga'[4] – much work of which was in fact carried out at the RFH! Wakefield will be remembered as the doctor who having failed to determine the aetiology of *Crohn's Disease* set about destruction of the concept of immunisation; he was also one of the first 'anti-vaxxers'.

I now include some reminiscences as one of the first *male* graduates of this teaching hospital and medical school which has now taken its place amongst the 'greats' such as St Thomas's and Guy's, etc, which for centuries had adorned the London medical scene (*see above*).

From then on my focus was on Hunter Street, Brunswick Square, and the *Royal Free Hospital School of Medicine* (the Dean of which at that time was an anaesthetist – Katharine Lloyd-Williams) – on the corner of the square and Handel Street. I was to attend this building almost daily from 1951 to 55 – a district of which had been made famous by the Bloomsbury Group (which included Virginia Woolf [1882-1941]) of the early 20th century, one of Charles Dickens (1812-70)'s houses, and the site of the Foundling Hospital (1739-

1926).*¹ 8 Hunter Street (home at that time of the RFH Medical School) always proved a friendly, almost 'family' setting and I invariably felt at home there.

Male students, who were then much in the minority (*see below*), always sat in close proximity to one another, at the rear of various lecture theatres, and at the back and upper left-hand corner – facing the lecturer. Several male students had previously graduated from the *RFHMS* since 1947 – Dowling Monroe, Brian Day, David Roberts and Michael Day are names coming to mind; so I was by no means the *first* male student!

This was a time of great change in London's practice of Medicine, all medical schools being compelled to take both sexes, there being only two in those days! (a move which did not go down well with most medical schools), and further the NHS was about to replace the longstanding *medical profession* which had been built up over many centuries. Among my *male* contemporaries were:

- *Lionel Boxall* – from Ilford, Essex (who became a dermatologist in Canada and had previously married a RFH nurse) – who I was to meet many years later.

- *Andrew Crowcroft* – who had already obtained a BSc in Psychiatry and was able to enlighten us on female sexual matters – including lesbianism.

- Paul Fursden – son of a Welsh Minister of Religion and an enthusiastic 'prankster' including: – a contribution of an 'unwelcome' addition to a batch of memorial plaques to commemorate previous 'lady' doctors trained at the *London School of Medicine for Women* (in the main quadrangle), a firework explosion during a lecture by Ruth Bowden (see below) and jam on the unveiling chord of a French portraitist. He was ultimately expelled from this medical school and became a dental student at Westminster Hospital. Many years later I was to meet him at the Society of Apothecaries of which I am a member.

- *John R M Gibson* – a talented 'rugger' player (a fullback) who was to play a great part in the early days of the RFH rugby team. He was also an excellent cricketer – an opening batsman I recall. I suspect, although I do not know, that Gibson had been educated at a *public* school, although

---

1. * London's first home for abandoned children – founded by the retired sea captain Thomas Coram (1668-1751) with a great deal of assistance from Georg Friedrich Händel (1685-1759) and later Dickens and William Hogarth (1697-1764). The hospital was relocated to Redhill, Surrey in 1926.

that was *not* a talking point in those days. I became secretary of both the rugby and cricket clubs. Incidentally, the RFH surgeon – George Qvist – was a tremendous and enthusiastic supporter of our rugger team.

- *Clive (Ronald) Kempster* – a former student of King's College School, Wimbledon, who was 'christened' by Fursden (*see above*) a 'goody'. He subsequently became an ophthalmic surgeon.

Also amongst close associates were Leila Liebster, Reg Rosser, and Peter Giles – who became a general practitioner. Incidentally, there were several portraits of distinguished pioneers of the history of 'women in medicine' in the Junior Common Room (JCR) – one of Sophia Jex-Blake (1846-1912), who Fursden (*see* above) insisted on referring to as 'Sex-Blake'; however, she was almost certainly a lesbian!

About that time the *NHS Act* had been passed – in 1946 in fact (one year after termination of World War II [1939-45] hostilities) and brought into action on 5 July 1948 (*see below*). It was thus a very exciting time for those of us who were by then well set to pursue a career in Medicine. Some of the undergraduates (*see above*) are indelibly preserved in my memory.

In all, there were some ten men and approximately eighty female undergraduates in the 1951 intake. This resulted, I recall, in conversion of the women's lavatories, with the men's now in the *new* block – in the cellar.

A common meeting point for the undergraduates was the *Junior Common Room* (JCR) *before* the 9.00am lectures – especially following weekends; one or another student would regale the others with their more interesting or exciting activities. Recollection of one woman's 'nightmare' comes to mind (I suppose because it was so unusual). She had been conveyed to a picnic party in the countryside and was desperate to urinate. However, she said she found this *impossible* without the usual domestic appliances; she considered this her personal 'inhibition'. This was the first time I had heard of this strange malady[2]*. She told her assembled audience that she was thus condemned to a distended bladder for the remainder of that day.

A favourite restaurant for 'afternoon tea' was one in Marchmont Street – a stone's throw from the Medical School. Then there were the 'domestic' staff: Mrs Brandreth (librarian), Miss Norfolk (refectory). But who were the pre-clinical lecturers? They are all included in the Annual Brochure of the medical school.

The dominant subject of study by far was *Anatomy*, and much of one's

---

2. * 'Shy-bladder syndrome' (paruresis) is apparently of psychiatric origin and overall more common in men than women.

time was occupied with dissection of the human body. Professor Ruth E M Bowden had recently been appointed to the *Chair of Anatomy* in succession to Mary Lucas-Keene and was very much in charge. Little was seen or heard from other members of the department – Michael Blunt and the Shattock family*[3]. Physiology was largely dealt with by several members of that department – Marjorie ('Daisy') Duckworth, Roland Moore, Brenda Ryman, and others, and Biochemistry by Frederick Kursner.

It was during this phase of my undergraduate career that the *Royal Free* and its branches were closed owing to outbreak of a 'mysterious' infection which came to become known as '*Royal Free Disease*' and now seems to have been a version of *Chronic Fatigue Syndrome*, although more work is needed to confirm this. I was then transferred with Paul Robert (from Switzerland) to St Olave's Hospital, Rotherhithe for Gynaecology in the Department of Miss Margaret Salmond.

A later development at this now bisexual school, was a sports ground. The authorities bought Middleton House near Enfield, Middlesex – which later had all necessary facilities for both men and women students, the latter sex frequently talking of 'lacs' presumably referring to lacrosse, of which I knew nothing at all, which at that time was apparently played at many girls' public schools.

The BSc Physiology course

I obtained excellent marks in examinations leading to the MB, BS degrees. The Professor of Physiology, Esther Margaret Killick (1902-6]) (whose husband was the Professor of Physiology at *St Mary's Hospital Medical School*) invited two members of the 1951 intake to undertake a BSc (special) degree course in the following eighteen months; they were Mary Underwood and myself. Two of those from other schools reading Physiology (London Hospital in this case) were: Peter Richardson**[4] and Tony Hicklin. This was a course based at several of London's medical schools and those I recall taking part were:

---

3   * Mr Shattock was a surgeon at the Royal Free, his wife a psychiatrist and their son – who worked in the Anatomy Department – was 'christened' by the female undergraduates – 'Baby Shatt'.

4   ** Richardson's wife was a daughter of the Anglican Bishop of Hong Kong, the name of whom I think was Hall. During WWII (1939-45); he is renowned for ordaining a woman owing to a sparsity of male recruits; this was of course against the rules of the Anglican Church, and he was severely reprimanded by the Archbishop of Canterbury of the time.

- *Middlesex* – Sampson Wright, A A G Lewis,
- *Guy's* – Professor Robson (Pharmacology),
- *'Bart's'* – Professor Rotblat,
- *St Thomas's* – Professor Henry Barcroft, FRS, and
- *King's College* – Professor R J S McDowell.

This went very well, Mary Underwood obtaining a first class (physiology) degree while I had to make do with an upper-second (two-one). These were days of course, when this country had far fewer universities than it does today; it also awarded far fewer first-class degrees than now. Where will it all end?

I also recall numerous visits both then and also in my pre-clinical years to a house in Keats Grove, Hampstead (near the Lawn Road branch of the RFH), which for a short time was occupied by the poet and medical student John Keats [1795-1821].[5]

References and notes

1. S Griffiths, H Yorke. British students locked out at new medical schools: despite high demand from UK applicants for places, universities can charge £45,000 a year for foreign applicants. *Sunday Times, Lond* 2022; 4 December: 6;. K Lay. Just two in five junior doctors now UK-trained. *Times, Lond* 2022 19 October: 10.
2. G C Cook. The Asiatic cholera: an historical determinant of human genomic and social structure. In: B S Drasar and B D Forest (eds). *Cholera and the ecology of Vibrio cholerae.* London: Chapman & Hall 1996: 18-53.
3. C Blake. *The Charge of the Parasols: women's entry to the Medical Profession.* London: The Women's Press Ltd. 1990:254; F Sandwith. *Surgeon Compassionate: the story of Dr William Marsden MD, MRCS.* London: Peter Davies 1960: 235; L A Amidon. *An Illustrated History of the Royal Free Hospital.* London: Special Trustees of the Royal Free Hospital 1996: 131; R Holmes. *Sylvia Pankhurst: natural born rebel.* Bloomsbury 2020: 976; K Lay. Health service too reliant on foreign nurses, says regulator. *Times, Lond* 2020; July 16.
4. B Deer. *The Doctor who fooled the world: Andrew Wakefield's war on vaccines.* London: Scribe 2020: 394. *See also*: I Yeomans. Universities tackle grade inflation by cutting firsts. *Times, Lond* 2022 5 July: 1.
5. L Miller. *Keats: a brief life in nine poems and one epitaph.* London: Penguin 2021: 358.

Chapter Three

Medical Training: II. Clinical

At this point – and with the BSc out of the way, it was time to re-join my original intake, resume my *clinical* studies and begin *clinical**[5] training. I had fallen 18 months behind my *original* intake – due to the BSc in physiology course – so I had to catch up with them and also get to know the following intake. Of course by the time I joined my former colleagues eighteen months had passed, but those of us who had taken the BSc course (*see* Chapter 2) were far more well- informed regarding human physiology, in particular history of haemoglobin research, but also knew how to use a library and/or write a medical paper. The next few years were then devoted to (i) completion of the *clinical* course leading to qualification in medicine, and (ii) obtaining employment, preferably at one's own teaching hospital or one in its group.

In those distant days, clinical teaching was *dominated* by 'George' and 'Fanny' (George Qvist FRCS and Dame Frances Gardner FRCP, Surgeon and Physician respectively to the *Royal Free*). Without them *clinical* teaching would have been sparse indeed. Apart from Qvist and Gardner, much of the teaching was undertaken by registrars or senior registrars.

All *clinical* teaching was enacted in old (mostly Victorian) buildings housing the Royal Free's extensions, and only a minority in the main edifice in Gray's Inn Road. Among members of the following intake were several potential doctors who I got to know well: Joe Hall and 'Fergie' (who I believe became

---

5   * Clinical originally meant 'bed-side' and had been used in that context since the ancient Greeks. Now that definition has been extended and is even used in numerous alternative ways, eg to describe a soccer goal in Britain's 'beautiful game'.

an orthopaedic surgeon, James Cope (who I had met on my first day at the medical school and who became a GP in the City of London, and died at the ripe old age of 90 years), 'Taffy' Jenkins – a most valuable member of our 'rugger' team – a hooker who was well versed with the tricks of that trade like any true Welshman. Then there was a rather older Indian – Nariman Bamji (1909-78) – who incidentally was a Parsee. And what of Lady Jane Bingham (sister of the notorious Lord Lucan [1934 – ?])[1] daughter of an earl and student in the 'new' intake?; I know she qualified but to where did she gravitate? The USA I believe, but I lack details.

As students we carefully followed the careers of 'George' and 'Fanny' intimately (they eventually became married!). George Qvist was to perform numerous operations on Frances Gardner's mitral stenotic patients. Mitral stenosis was of course commonly caused by *rheumatic fever* and was relatively common in those days. Another 'character' of those years was a physician – Una Ledingham – whose ward rounds often lasted 8 hours or more!

It was during those years that I also learned a lot about *infective* disease – Lawn Road previously being the North-west (of London) fever hospital in Victorian times. The infectious disease physicians were: 'Willy' Gunn and Melvyn Ramsay; the latter was to become fascinated by '*Royal Free disease*' which in 1955 had closed the Royal Free hospitals (*see above*), and now seems to be a form of *chronic fatigue syndrome* (*see above*)!

As far as I am aware, the 'Free' did *not* have an archivist in those days. I recall that a former *Royal Free* anaesthetist– Edith Gilchrist – once occupied the post. Now the material is I believe, accommodated at the London Metropolitan archive, Farringdon.

Clinical teaching was in all respects excellent – in those somewhat inadequate buildings of Victorian times which had been taken over by the NHS.

At the end of my *clinical* training years, I qualified with the MRCS, LRCP diplomas and the University of London degrees of MB and BS (*see* fig 1).

Opposite: Fig 1: Group of newly qualified junior doctors in 2023 – on strike for an increase in pay. **P Brookes. Times, Lond 2023; 21 September: 25 (Kind permission of The Times & Peter Brookes.)**

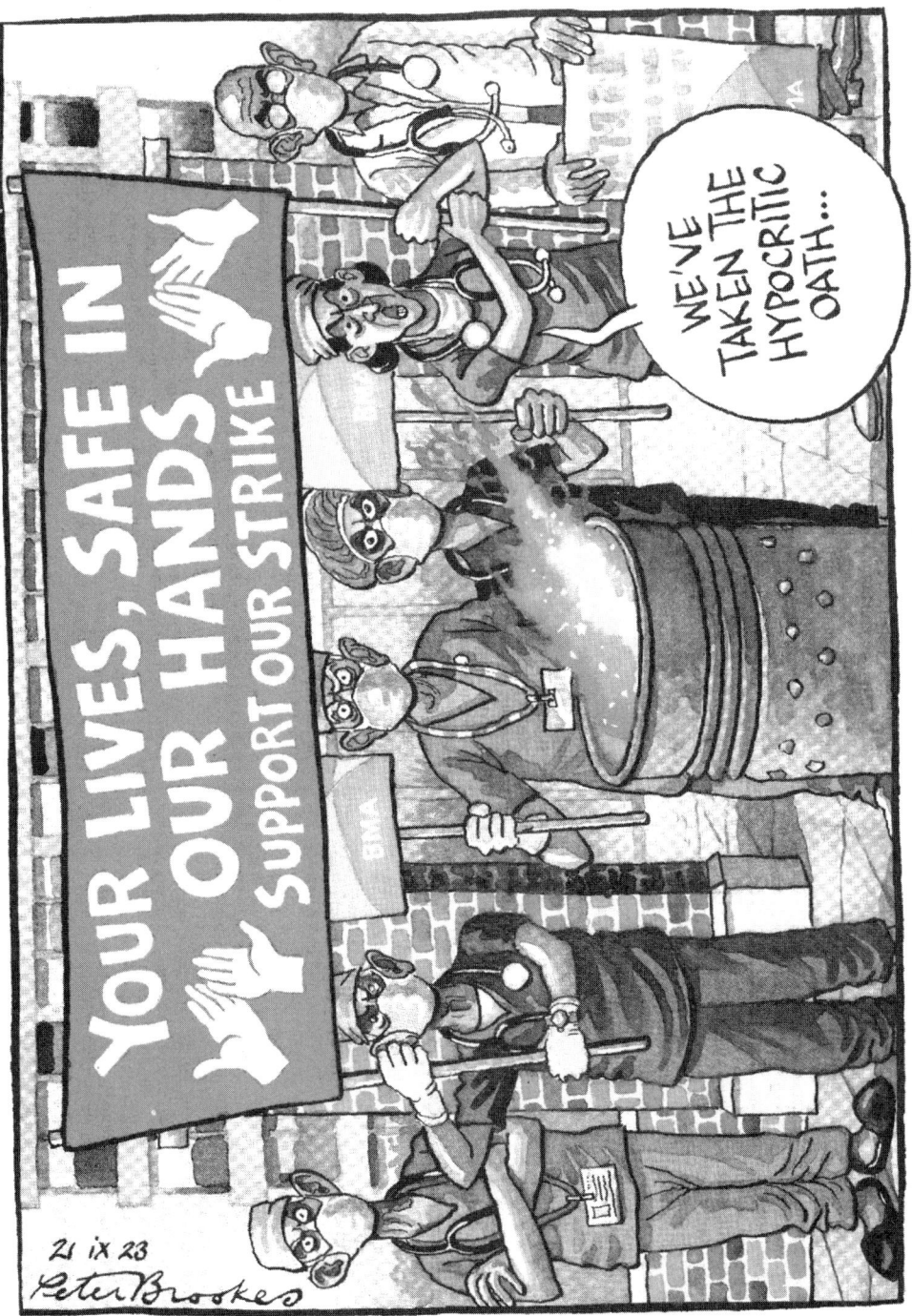

References

1. L Thompson. *A Different Class of Murder: the story of Lord Lucan.* London: Head of Zeus Ltd 2018: 431; C Wace. Colonel Mustard card discovery deepens Lucan murder mystery. *Times, Lond* 2022; 5 November: 8; R Kinchen. I will never stop looking for Lucan, my mum's murderer: when Neil Berriman, a Hampshire builder, discovered he was the son of Sandra Rivett, the nanny killed by Lord Lucan, an obsessive search began. Fifteen years on, completely new clues emerged. *Sunday Times, Lond* 2022; 13 November: 22; A Vaux. Nine-day queen given a new lease of life. *Times, Lond* 2022 27 December: 11.

Chapter Four

The pre-registration years

Before one was 'let loose' in those days on Britain's population it was essential to complete at least two 'House' appointments.

House appointments

Following a *locum* appointment at the **Princess Alice Hospital, Eastbourne**, it was time to begin my four proper pre-registration appointments. Financial reward was certainly not a priority in those days; writing from memory, I seem to recall an annual salary of £452 to cover 'board and lodging'.

After attending numerous ward-rounds with (Dame) Frances Gardner as a clinical student, she accepted me as her House Physician at the **Lawn Road branch of RFH**. The emphasis was on cardiology and I particularly recall the cardiac catheter sessions at Lawn Road – on Thursday mornings – when the Countess of Lucan, a distinguished biochemist in her own right, was always on duty! These were the days of anticoagulants following a myocardial infarction, and Gardner had an obsession that the injection had to be administered precisely *on time* – day or night! This clearly absorbed a great deal of my time and energy; as a result however I knew almost every inch of the corridors of the former North-west fever hospital.[1] The other consultant physician on that 'firm' was Nigel Compston CBE, later to play a major rôle in creation of the *new* RFH at Hampstead – erected on the site of the Lawn Road hospital.

My next employment was at **Hampstead General Hospital** (Royal Free group), where I was to work for three consultants: Cameron McLeod, Emlyn Williams, and Joseph Minton, all surgeons. *Mr Cameron McLeod* FRCS was the senior surgeon. He was a graduate of St Mary's Hospital and his brother had been appointed to their Chair of Obstetrics; in fact, Cameron was the 'failed' member of his generation – a proud man who only performed relatively minor operations; I got on well with him. *Emlyn Williams* FRCS was a gastroenterological surgeon, specialising in colonic surgery. He allowed me freedom in administration of, for example, post-operative intravenous fluids, and by following a book written by the Middlesex surgeon – Leslie Lequesne – I was able to 'manage' the post-operative course of his patients. Williams was a heavy smoker and at one stage during my employment he was suspected of having a bronchial carcinoma (which fortunately transpired not to be the case). Minton was an ophthalmic surgeon and I well recall applying leeches (*Hirudo medicinalis*) to his patients with glaucoma.

Having now held junior appointments in medicine *and* surgery, I felt that one in pathology might be appropriate, so I applied for and was duly appointed to a position at the now extinct **Royal Northern Hospital** in Holloway Road. *Michael Peters* was in charge of post-mortems for north London and I was destined to carry out many of these; there was a highly experienced technician from whom I learned much – not only in gross anatomy, but also in histological matters. *Martin Hynes* was the other consultant pathologist, although he occupied most of his time in private practice at Harley Street. My major contact with him was cross-matching of blood for transfusion; I think he relied on my services at night when most laboratories were closed; Hynes I recall always paid me for my services. Although the Royal Northern had, and in the past had had many individuals of distinction on its staff list, I met only a few. In the past, *Robert Bridges* – a former poet laureate, had served as a physician at that hospital. There was Raymond Greene – brother of Graham (the author), and Carleton and (Sir) Reginald Murley – who rightly in my opinion vigorously opposed introduction of the NHS in its final form, and Gabriel the colorectal surgeon (known to all and sundry as the 'Arse-Angel' Gabriel).

Following these three House jobs, I was to move to the **(Royal) Brompton Hospital** where my 'chiefs' were (Sir) Kenneth Robson FRCP (*St George's* and later Registrar of the *Royal College of Physicians*) and Howard Nicholson FRCP (*University College*). I also had the privilege of contact with Russell Brock (later Lord Brock of Wimbledon), Paul Wood (cardiologist), Clement Price-Thomas (who performed the King's pneumonectomy), Matthew Paneth and 'Pasty' Barrett. But my time at the Brompton was mildly complicated – three months at the Brompton Sanatorium (the superintendent being Dr Aylmer Foster-Carter); tuberculosis was still a common infection in Britain, and then six months as house physician and resident assistant medical officer at the Brompton Hospital itself.

These were halcyon days, most hospitals mentioned having now been demolished. During these appointments I had applied for and been successful in postponing *National Service*. But now I could delay it no longer! I chose to contribute not to the *RAMC* – to which I had been recruited – but to the *Royal Nigerian Army* (RNA), most of my service taking place at Lagos, Nigeria.

References and notes

1. *See* ref 2 Chapter 2 (Amidon: 1996).

Chapter Five

AFTER NATIONAL SERVICE – 1962 ONWARDS

These two years proved to be my introduction to *clinical tropical medicine* – the *colonial* discipline created by Sir Patrick Manson in 1899. I saw a great deal of *malaria*, *schistosomiasis*, and *tuberculosis* in Nigerian soldiers. I had attended a few formal lectures by Alan Woodruff during my student days, but the *clinical* component was then missing. These two years are described in an autobiography, and were the introduction to my subsequent career.[1]

At this juncture I had thus committed myself to a discipline with which I did not seriously believe! It was all very well in the early *twentieth* century, when Harley Street practitioners knew little of disease in tropical countries, but by the 1960s this was not necessarily the case.

Having completed *National Service* in 1962 it was obviously time to obtain civilian employment. I was fortunate in that a physician with whom I had worked at the Brompton – Robson – suggested that I might be interested in a registrar post for the following year at **St George's Hospital** (Tooting branch), with James Dow, which I was delighted to take. Dow was one of the old school of gastroenterologists so, as well as *tropical medicine,* I was able to add *gastroenterology* to my curriculum vitae. Although I later joined the *British Society of Gastroenterology* my ambition was always to be a *general* physician of whom there are abysmally few at present; 'a*s regular as clockwork*' was a phrase I was to hear frequently in relation to 'bowel activity' in my subsequent career as a gastroenterologist. But of course *clockwork* has now been overtaken by the conglomeration of devices known as the internet, so such phrases are alas things of the past! Most of my time was spent at St George's, Tooting branch; this was before the hospital transferred there, with a weekly outpatient session at Hyde Park Corner. One of my minor 'hobbies' at St George's was a weekly MRCP introductory course designed to assist candidates pass the MRCP examination, most attending an ongoing course by a man named Maurice Papworth. One memorable but sad event at St George's was that the house-physician on Dow's firm decided to commit suicide; he was Jewish and apparently simply could not cope with the duties of house-physician!

A year is a relatively short time not only in politics, and my next move was therefore an important one. So far, I had had no exposure to *academic* medicine, but began a post as lecturer with Professor (Dame) Sheila Sherlock FRCP at the **Royal Free** – my original teaching hospital.

In my absence abroad things had moved fast at the '*Free*'; *academic* medicine had been introduced and the old stalwarts, led by Gardner had lost the battle. Academic medicine had at last been introduced and a 'hut' on a roof of the hospital had been erected for this purpose.

Sherlock's unit was largely built around her. It was confined to this wooden hut on the roof of the old RFH, which in fact served as its 'home' until the move to the new building at Hampstead (*see above*). The 'second in command' was Tony Dawson (1928-97]) (later to become Sir Anthony, physician to HM the Queen). Barbara Billing later became a personal professor although *not* medically qualified. Then there were numerous research fellows – mostly from the USA. Among the British fellows were: Neil McIntyre, Geoffrey Walker, Jonathan Levy and Roger Williams.[2] Of the USA contributors, I remember many but since most remained for short periods only, it is difficult to recall their names. Although the emphasis was on *liver disease* and its complications, Sherlock was very conscious that other systems must also be covered.

Personally, my major interests were initially with hepatotoxins and conduction of a 'controlled' trial of corticosteroids in *active chronic hepatitis* (a term which incidentally was criticised by amongst others 'Fanny' Gardner, who argued that no process could be both active *and* chronic). Lectures and discussion meetings took place at regular intervals and I learned a great deal about *academic* medicine and more specifically liver disease. Overall, this was a most valuable two years but I missed the 'tropics' and its diseases enormously; when an advertisement appeared in both the *Lancet* and *British Medical Journal* (BMJ) for a lecturer in medicine at *Makerere University College* (later Makerere University), Kampala, Uganda I immediately applied and was appointed.

The Renowned Makerere University College, Uganda

This episode in my medical career lasted from mid 1965 until mid 1967. As a lecturer at Makerere, I practised clinical medicine at the Mulago Hospital and carried out research at the *Medical Research Council's Child Nutrition Unit*. The latter proved to be extremely productive from my personal viewpoint (in 1966 two first papers in the *Lancet* were published: one on *lactase* in the indigenous population) propelled me into the international academic field! Incidentally, subsequent discussion about *lactase* and milk consumption evolutionarily probably led to the acceptance of importance of *vitamin D* and its relation to immunity and possibly dementia. My work on *lactase* is summarised in a book – *The Milk Enzyme*.

The first of these investigations demonstrated that while most thoroughbred Ugandan Africans had hypolactasia in adult life, those from tribes from northern Africa and/or the middle-east (although also black-skinned) had persistent *lactase* (PL) in adult life like most white-skinned Europeans and their *descendants*. The leading hypothesis for these findings was that a mutation had occurred in the *lactase* gene when *Homo sapiens* left Africa for Europe and Asia, which generated a survival advantage. While this might have conveyed multiple advantages, widespread immunity resulting from vitamin D deficiency might have been one of these. Recent research on this vitamin in sufferers of Alzheimer's, dementia and other cognitive disorders *might* have been one of these.[3]

This continuation of my 'tropical' experience increased my realisation that there were numerous 'medical' problems 'out there' to be solved; and what were those in medicine (like me) doing? We were sitting in a developed and wealthy Britain while former colonies were inundated with problems which should have been solved many years earlier. Justin Welby (105th *Archbishop of Canterbury*) has concluded that the *British Empire* was totally corrupt, but the late Archbishop of York – black-skinned and born in Uganda – held a very different view! Anyway, it was at this stage that I decided to devote more time to medicine in third-world countries.

Following Uganda, it was back to London where with the help of others I completed the controlled trial of corticosteroids in *active chronic hepatitis* and which was published in the then prestigious *Quarterly Journal of Medicine*. Back in Sherlock's department, I resumed where I had left off. I also became absorbed with investigation of refined-sucrose (sugar); several allied projects related to fructose (a component of sucrose) and I concluded that this was probably the 'toxic' component of sucrose causing obesity, although not everyone was in agreement (*see* fig 2). This work was published in *Clinical Science*, a leading clinical/physiological journal. I was progressing with my sucrose research when an advertisement for a Professor of Medicine (and *not*

METABOLIC RESEARCH LABORATORY

From
H. A. Krebs

NUFFIELD DEPARTMENT OF CLINICAL MEDICINE

Radcliffe Infirmary,
Oxford.

Tel. Oxford 49891, Ext. 244

OX2 6HE

25th February, 1969.

Dr. G.C. Cook,
Department of Medicine,
The Royal Free Hospital,
Gray's Inn Road,
London, W.C.1.

Dear Dr. Cook,

I am afraid I cannot offer really useful comments on your preliminary data on fructose metabolism in man. Similar work has been carried out in several centres (see for example Tygstrup et al., J.Clin.Invest. 47, 817, 1967; Heinz et al., J.Clin.Invest. 47, 1826, 1968; Zalatis & Oliver, Biochem.J. 107, 753, 1967; Zöllner, Klin.Woch., 46, 1300, 1968). However the suggestion that there may be two different kinds of population is certainly new and interesting. It is not likely that there are two major pathways of fructose metabolism. It seems to be more probable that the differences which you notice are due to quantitative variations.

It is certainly possible to assay the key enzymes of fructose metabolism on human liver biopsy specimens. My colleague, L.V. Eggleston, has recently carried out such assays on rat liver samples. He used relatively large quantities of tissue but I believe the methods could be adapted to smaller samples. Should you be interested in these assays I should be glad to supply full particulars. Most of the necessary information is contained, or referred to, in the publications mentioned above.

Yours sincerely,

H.A. Krebs.

Fig 2: Letter from the foremost expert on fructose metabolism (Professor H A Krebs FRS) during my research spell on sucrose at the Department of Medicine, the Royal Free Hospital School of Medicine.

the head of healthcare services) at the relatively *new* University in Lusaka, Zambia (formerly Northern Rhodesia) appeared in the medical journals; I duly applied and was interviewed at the Inter-University's Council by Lord (Max) Rosenheim – recently retired president of the *Royal College of Physicians of London* – and the Dean of the London Hospital Medical College, and to my astonishment was appointed (see fig 3). This was a *new* school whilst the Old *Lusaka Central Hospital* – which had opened in colonial times (in the 1930s) – was by then hopelessly inadequate and out-of-date.

Many times I have wondered exactly (especially by the 'man in the street') what the population of Zambia, and Lusaka in particular really expected their updated medical facilities to be? He/she probably anticipated an exact replacement for his/her *old* hospital – built some half-century ago – and staff to go with it; instead they had to accept the *new* UTH, a university hospital with *academic* staff and facilities; was this what they wanted? What did *academic* mean anyway? This was a stressful and extremely busy five years, outlined in an unpublished book which dealt with that subject.

The people of Lusaka were unlike Africans I had previously known and worked with in Nigeria and Uganda, the black/white issue (in southern Africa) – apartheid and colonisation both being highly prominent and emotive topics. Early months were occupied with compilation of teaching timetables for introductory lectures etc; it had not yet been decided what sort of medical school and curriculum was contemplated. I was soon to find that medical facilities had been so neglected in recent years that even the Zambian *Minister of Health* was sceptical of the *new University Teaching Hospital* (UTH). Many times I had stressed to both staff and students the importance of *clinical* research in this new facility; my personal research results are recorded in the *Appendix.* I chose the effect of systemic infection on ingested foodstuffs as my major research theme. Of course there were other topics also, including the *lactase* issue (*see above*). I understand that retrospectively certain individuals (including the first graduates of the Zambian school) used the *colonial* and *apartheid* issues to suggest that my *primary* reason for going to Zambia for five years was to 'experiment' on black-skinned people because I couldn't find suitable volunteers in Britain (this was a story much later accepted without any evidence by future employers – including Woodruff and the Dean of the 'LSHTM') and that altruism was merely a figment of my imagination! Nothing could have been further from the truth, and was obviously damaging to my future career; posterity might sort this out but individuals in this part of Africa, it must be accepted, had an enormous 'chip on the shoulder'.

A Life in Medicine : a British Doctor's Account

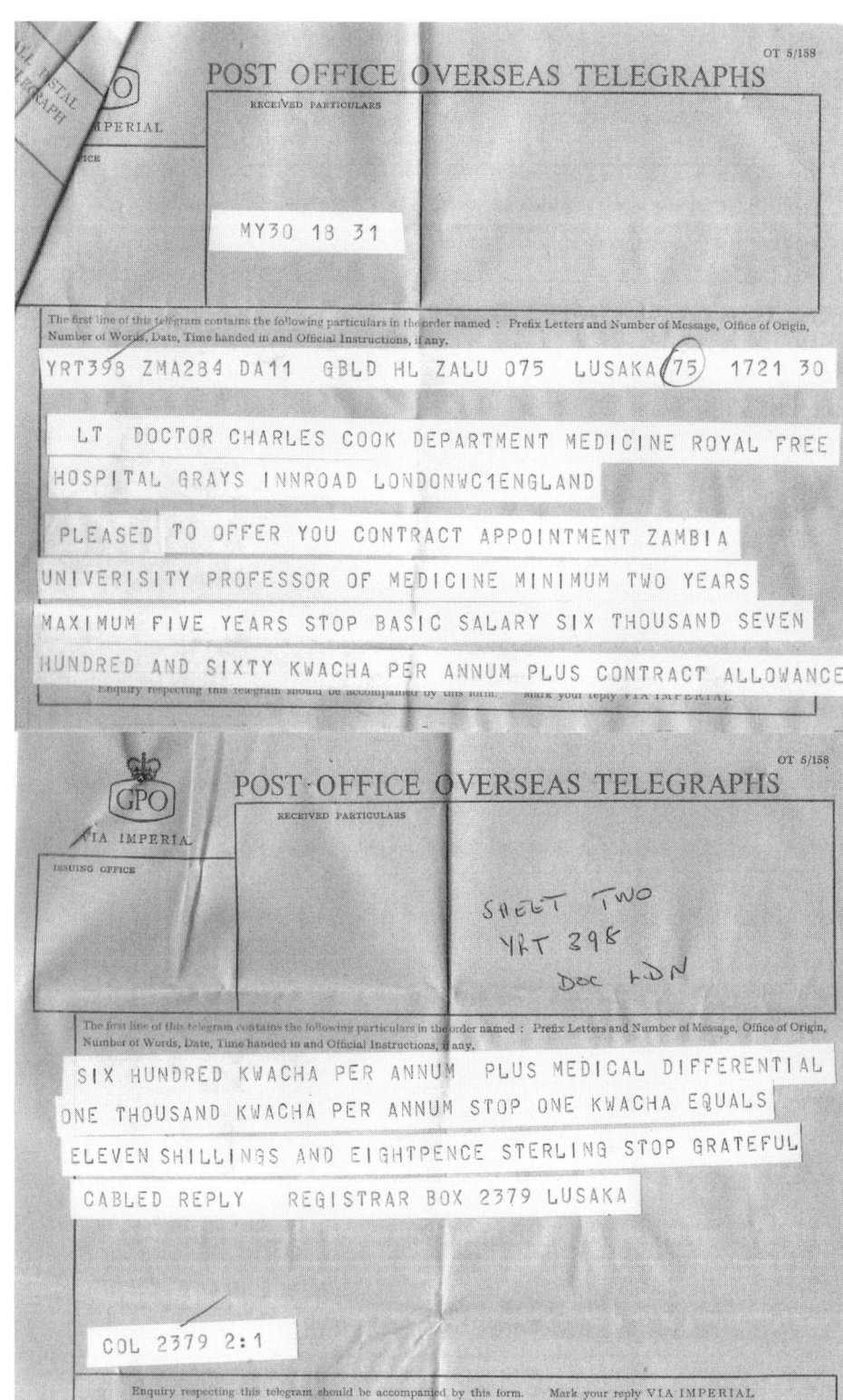

One of my greatest disappointments in Zambia came towards the end of my stay, when my much anticipated external examiner for the first *final* examination suddenly and unexpectedly died (*see* fig 4). Professor Lord Rosenheim (1908-72) was apparently looking forward to going to Lusaka when he suddenly developed a dissecting aortic aneurism which killed him. Rosenheim had recently retired from the presidency of the *Royal College of Physicians of London* and this left me in a particularly difficult situation.

PROFESSOR LORD ROSENHEIM

Home Address:-
39 ETON AVENUE,
LONDON, N.W.3.
01- 794 3320

UNIVERSITY COLLEGE HOSPITAL,
LONDON. W.C.1.
01- 387 9300

22nd April 1972

Professor G. C. Cook,
School of Medicine,
The University of Zambia,
P.O. Box 2379, Lusaka, ZAMBIA.

Dear Professor Cook,

Thank you very much for your letter of April 13th. and for the most pleasant invitation to come out as the External Examiner at your first final examination in Medicine next January.

I feel very honoured at being asked and am most grateful to the Vice-Chancellor and yourself. I should be delighted to come out and should prefer the first week - January 15th to 20th. As you know I visited Lusaka for a few days in 1969 and I look forward to seeing the changes that have taken place since then. I have been very interested in the Medical School since it started.

I am delighted that Council has put your name forward for the Fellowship. This is so very well deserved and I send you my warmest congratulations. I ceased to be President at the end of March, after six years, and have been succeeded by Cyril Clarke, Professor of Medicine at Liverpool. I am very glad that he is following me. I am gradually getting used to "civilian" life again.

I look forward to January and to seeing you, though you may appear in June for admission. If so, let us have a chat.

All good wishes and very many thanks,

Yours sincerely,

Fig. 3: *The telegram offering the Chair of Medicine in the* University of Zambia *to the author.*

Fig 4: *Letter from Lord Rosenheim FRCP, FRS to Lusaka in which he expressed his great pleasure at being invited to be external examiner in the first final examination in Medicine in the* University of Zambia.

After my 5-year contract had expired, so productive had my research been in Uganda and Zambia that I decided to submit my papers for a DSc in the *University of London*; this proved successful and I am thus a holder of one of the University's *major* awards – the DSc degree.

Over these five years in Lusaka I had worked probably harder than either before or since. Now that most 'third-world' countries possess their own university and medical school, it seems unlikely that an expatriate *professor of medicine* will be required in the future at any of Britain's former possessions anyway; I suppose the younger generation and members of the 'black lives matter' movement will see to that. Incidentally, when they realise that evolutionarily we were once all black-skinned and that *white* men/women are the 'abnormal' ones following a colour mutation, they *might* have second thoughts!

It was difficult to decide where to head for next. I was offered employment at several 'tropical' medical schools, but was ultimately attracted to one in **Riyadh, Saudi Arabia**, sponsored by the *University of London*. However, on arrival I soon found out that this was in a *very* early stage of development, and also that the Islamic male/white barrier to mixed sex teaching meant that instruction, which I had successfully carried out in Lusaka, was impossible. Also it had *not* been decided exactly where teaching would take place; following negotiations to which I was not privy it was finally decided that a former small, *private* hospital – the *Abdul Aziz* – was satisfactory for this purpose. However, I thought otherwise and therefore I (and my family) left Riyadh after one university year. In fact, the *Abdul Aziz* Hospital was fit for only *minor* illnesses and I thus failed to obtain a true picture of disease in Riyadh, although it was obvious that obesity and all its resultant problems was a massive issue – undoubtedly a result of a huge intake of refined-sucrose (sugar) in the local diet. But I had extended the *lactase* story on which I did some research and wrote a short paper which the *BMJ* kindly published (*see The Milk Enzyme*).

This latter instalment of my *itinerant* career was particularly unfortunate; I suspect I was not made fully aware of numerous problems of Riyadh by their London representative – 'Teddy' Johnson – my hope of remaining in Riyadh for several years were thus scuppered! Now, I was unemployed again! I continued to be sceptical that the *outdated* discipline (tropical medicine) still existed, and in consequence my future in medicine was made even more complicated.

(Sir) Graham Bull was aware that Britain's *Medical Research Council* (MRC) was looking for a successor to Murray Baker to fill the '*tropical medicine*' slot at their headquarters office; this I filled for the next few months. While I was working at the MRC headquarters, I received what transpired to be an important telephone call from Professor Alan Woodruff, Director of the *clinical* department of the *London School of Hygiene and Tropical Medicine* (LSHTM)*[5], asking if I would like to apply for a senior lectureship in his department because Clinton Manson-Bahr (grandson of Sir Patrick Manson – *see above*) had resigned in order to spend more time writing the next edition of *Manson's Tropical Diseases*. This seemed to me an ideal 'offer' which would both heal my financial concerns and seal my future as a *tropical medicine* physician; after all, who was more well qualified than me to fill this post? I sought the opinion of Tony Bryceson (1934-2023) who at that time was dividing his practice between private practice and London's *Hospital for Tropical* Diseases (HTD), who I found very encouraging. Both Woodruff and the Dean of that school (Dr C E Gordon Smith) assured me that I would soon be appointed to either a readership and/or personal chair; the latter said I might have to '*wait a few months in order to be fair to my colleagues*'.

At this point I had, looking back, made what was almost certainly the worst decision of my medical career!

I soon discovered what a 'fraud' Woodruff was – he had no library or laboratory in his department and one was expected to serve as his personal house-physician. In addition he had *zero* facilities for clinical research. Meanwhile, the Dean told me personally that he did not consider that the *clinical* department should actually exist in his *School of Hygiene* (I don't think he ever visited the HTD). Promises were never fulfilled and I remain amazed that these two senior individuals were so overtly dishonest in their behaviour!

---

5   * This wholly inadequate, inward-looking 'snobby' individual had occupied the Wellcome Chair at the LSHTM for some 30 years in the now extinct discipline of Tropical Medicine. His overriding contribution was preservation of his Directorship, for which he was not qualified in any way! During that time also, his sole academic contribution to the discipline had been to the incidence of the parasite *Toxocara canis* in Britain's public parks! His legacy has therefore faded into oblivion and insignificance beside the numerous distinguished contributions from his predecessors, the pioneers of the discipline which included Sir Patrick Manson and Sir Neil Hamilton-Fairley. Like Smith (the LSHTM's Dean) he made all personal and departmental decisions on 'political' and certainly not academic criteria. Another of Woodruff's ploys was to keep patients with a trivial illness in hospital for as long as possible in order to keep his bed occupancy raised; this resulted in the HTD being known as the: Hôtel Tropicale!

But nevertheless, I served as one of Woodruff's 'house physicians' in the meantime, and it was at least productive for my bank balance, because having served abroad for several years this was at that time in a most unsatisfactory state. Had I not been so altruistic in my early career, I would probably have been in such a favourable financial position that I could resign from Woodruff's department, but this was not the case.

I subsequently applied for several alternative jobs, but the 'rat-race in Britain was/is so tight' that to switch from one discipline to another was virtually impossible. The vast majority of medically qualified individuals under whom I have worked during my medical career have been extremely decent people; two notable exceptions were thus the 'Director' of the *Hospital for Tropical Diseases* and the Dean of the *London School of Hygiene* to which the sub-title *Tropical Medicine* had later been added. To my mind neither should have occupied the position which they did.

Papua New Guinea (PNG)

By 1978 I was so utterly fed up with Woodruff's hopeless 'department' and the fact that he had no idea what *academic* medicine was, that I decided to take a few years out, and when the Chair of Medicine at Port Moresby, **Papua New Guinea** was advertised, I immediately applied and was appointed. PNG medicine was dominated by Australians – led by John Biddulph – who sought to inflict the teaching of 'revisionists' (*see* Appendix) and *not* that of orthodox practitioners – on the population of PNG: *Doctors for PNG* or *Doctors for the world;* with an Australian orientation, *'practitioners for PNG'* was already in the process of implementation. I thought otherwise and thus 'clashed' with the antipodean regime. I found this exercise instructive but, as I predicted, disaster was 'waiting in the wings'. Nevertheless I learned much about PNG medicine, and was again appalled at the dominance of *tuberculosis* which remains a major disease in every developing country in which I have worked, but has been largely eliminated from most *developed* countries. Thus, the concept of *tropical medicine* is seriously flawed; it is a discipline involving 'exotic' infections of the tropics which can be localised geographically – disease in the tropics is similar in every location worldwide and is dominated by *tuberculosis*. In PNG for example textbooks would have one believe that *Kuru* was a common entity, but working in Port Moresby for three years, I never saw a case! But PNG is 'Aussie' territory, and the 'Pom' as far as they are concerned is extremely unwelcome. As far as the *local* population is concerned however, the British doctor and his/her contribution is greatly valued. So by and large my stay in PNG was valued by Papua New Guineans but wholeheartedly opposed by Australians. From a personal point of view there is much to be said for welcoming wants of poorer sections of the community, while any attempt at altruism is distorted by the Aussie and used against one!

What next? I reluctantly resumed my humble job in Woodruff's department with absolutely no indication that he or Smith would recommend me for a University title! Woodruff was rarely to be seen at St Pancras anyway (*see my book on the history of LSHTM*); he was more likely to be found at the *Athenaeum Club* or travelling overseas performing a service known only to himself. Regrettably, this was the only *clinical* department of *tropical medicine* in England, the sole competitor being the *Liverpool* school. What, therefore, could be done for the remainder of one's active career?[4]

Postscript

While working at the *Hospital for Tropical Diseases* I saw numerous patients who had returned from a tropical country with *chronic fatigue syndrome*, which seemed to me similar to *Royal Free Disease* (*see* Chapter 2) although my colleagues were of the opinion that it had a psychiatric origin. At the time I favoured a tropical virus or possibly the antimalarial drug – Mefloquine[5] – as its cause.

After a great deal of thought I decided that things in Woodruff's department were so unlikely to improve research-wise, that I abandoned the idea of resuming research and was only left with *writing, and* therefore subsequently wrote numerous books on the *history* of medicine, that of the tropics in particular. Meanwhile, the sum total of research in *clinical* medicine to emerge from Woodruff's department after thirty years was *zero*. I sent copies of my books on the history of LSHTM (*see above*) to the current Dean and the editor of the *Lancet* and did *not* even receive a letter of acknowledgement or thanks from either. What is the LSHTM and the medical world coming to? Unless the LSHTM has recently made significant changes and introduced *academic* medicine to its *clinical* department, I most strongly recommend that anyone with a *clinical* orientation should avoid the LSHTM. I subsequently formed a far better relationship with the *Department of Infectious Diseases* at University College, London.

Long after *compulsory* retirement, the Covid-19 pandemic occurred and medical direction then took place from a government which knew little or nothing about management of any viral disease.

In concluding this chapter, and with a wholly unsatisfactory state of medicine in Britain, I remain uncertain as to whether I originally made a correct career choice. My initial intention was to become a zoologist and this priority – with a quarter of England's mammals facing extinction – suggests I might well have been correct!

References

1. G C Cook. *National Service fifty years ago: life of a medical conscript in West Africa.* St Albans: Tropzam 2014: 169.
2. Anonymous. Professor Roger Williams; leading liver specialist who worked on Europe's first transplant and found himself in the spotlight when George Best was his patient. *Times, Lond* 2020; 21 July: 49.
3. G C Cook. S K Kajubi. Tribal incidence of lactase-deficiency in Uganda. *Lancet* 1966 725-30; G C Cook. *The Milk Enzyme; adventures with the human lactase polymorphism.* Cambridgeshire; Melrose Books 2017: 118; T Whipple. Why a lucky few may help the rest of us beat disease. *Times, Lond* 2022; 26 December: 16; K Shea *et al.* Brain vitamin D forms, cognitive decline, and neuropathology in community-dwelling older adults. *Alzheimer's & Dementia* 202: 7-8
4. G C Cook. *Origin of a Medical Speciality: the Seamen's Hospital Society and tropical medicine.* St Albans: Tropzam 2012: 182; G C Cook. *The rise and fall of a medical specialty: London's clinical tropical medicine.* St Albans: Tropzam 2014: 129.
5. G C Cook. Malaria prophylaxis: Mefloquine toxicity should limit its use to treatment alone. *Br med J* 1995; 311: 190-1
6. N Badshah. Biodiversity crisis 'could threaten human existence'. *Times, Lond* 2022; 12 July: 2; A Vaughan: 200 countries to thrash out new deal for saving wildlife. *Ibid* 2022; 5 December: 5; A Vaughan. A blueprint to protect biodiversity. *Ibid* 2022; 20 December: 4; A Vaughan. Nations seal deal to preserve the natural world. *Ibid* 2022; 20 December:1; Anonymous. Saving nature: global agreement on protecting species and habitats is vital and welcome. *Ibid* 20 December: 32; R Blakely. Grumpy animals are having their grievances heard. *Ibid* 2022; 26 December: 13; T Whipple. Cutting-edge plan to nurture nature. *Ibid* 2022; 27 December: 10; Anonymous. Insect Interests. Beating young oak trees is a sensitive measure of conservation. *Ibid* 27 December: 27; W Humphries. Squirrelpox could wipe out our rare reds. *Ibid* 2023: 5 January: 14; R Blakely. Plea to save Madagascan wildlife that would take 23 million years to replace. *Ibid* 2023; 11 January: 14.

Overleaf: Fig 5: Britain was at that time afflicted by numerous strikes for an increase in pay, with widespread implications. **P Brookes. Times, Lond 2023: 2 September: 23. (Kind permission of The Times & Peter Brookes.)**

A Life in Medicine : a British Doctor's Account

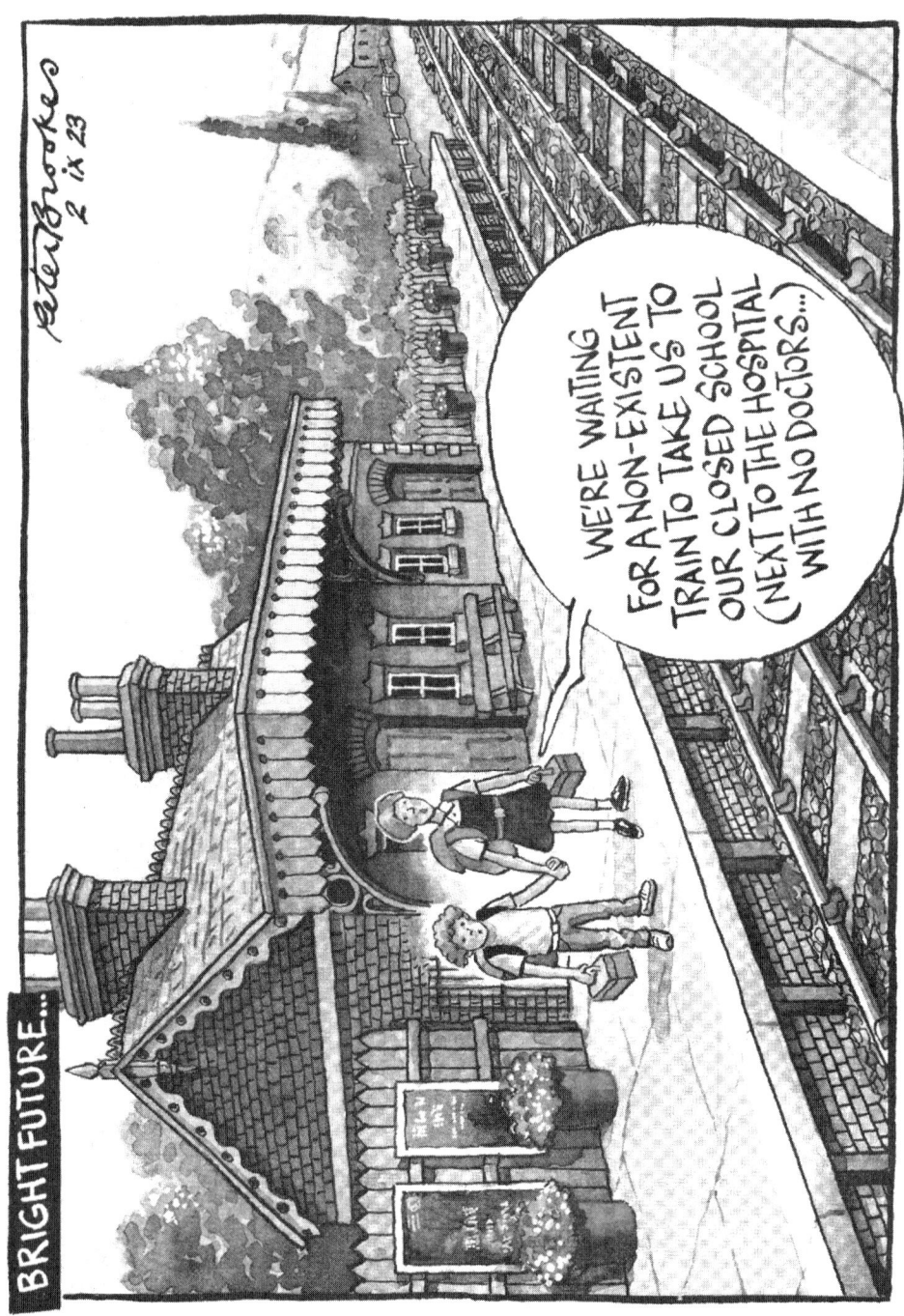

Epilogue

During the 1990s I became aware that the NHS (the *'free'* healthcare system run by politicians and *not* the medical profession) was functioning far less than satisfactorily. I propose therefore to quote examples of this but a solution is outside the scope of this book! Plans to take healthcare in this country away from the medical profession and make it a *political* pursuit were in preparation by the end of World War II (1939-45) under Clement Attlee (1853-1967)'s future Labour government; then in 1946 the *National Health Service* (NHS) *Act* was actually revealed and revised healthcare was launched two years later. Medicine in Britain was to be *free* for all and in the hands of politicians who knew little (if anything) about medicine.[1] Yes it would be free but was it right to place this highly specialised 'art' in the hands of untrained politicians? All went more or less well for the first half century, and the politicians merely gloated over their new-found vote-winner, while medical professionals watched in amazement; for the first time in recorded history, they had been relegated to that of government 'slaves'. British headlines in two respectable newspapers in 2022 (much later) summarising the position read: 'It's no longer feasible to be a full-time GP' and 'Ruinous bullying and sexism push NHS vacancies to 105,000'. Surely Britain *must* have a healthcare system which is superior to this! The *Sunday Times* pronounced in an editorial: 'No more task forces: the NHS crisis calls for tough decisions; please give healthcare in Britain back to where it belongs, it can't do worse than this'. In addition, 40 new hospitals were promised, but none of these had even been started at the time of writing.

All medical graduates after 1948 inevitably lived under the NHS regime; thus I have been compulsorily employed under this system whilst in Britain for by far the major part of my active medical career. As my career unfolded, I had increasingly wondered what a '*doctor*' was; he/she now differs so much from the 'doctor' of my childhood days (*see* above) that I just wonder whether we require a new title? To me the first doctors that I can recall (now defunct) were *friendly* general practitioners (GPs) while 'specialists' (then few and distant) were separate and far away (*see also* ref 1). Now we have a bunch of government servants or 'slaves', some being vaguely reminiscent of the old GP, although totally without an individualistic approach, and the 'specialist', who although initially trained to be a GP, could not possibly practise as one. Also, should the courtesy title 'doctor' still apply to all?

From a personal viewpoint I have enjoyed my career in medicine apart from the unfortunate time at the HTD and LSHTM (the Woodruff years). To make matters worse, the then Dean of the LSHTM (under whom the HTD lay) told me that the *clinical* department did *not* fit his *School of Hygiene* (*see above*). Woodruff was a most inappropriate individual to head any *academic* establishment at any time.

Change(s) to medical practice since the 1930s

Medicine as a discipline in Britain has been evolving for thousands of years. Changes in general practice particularly, occurred during the *industrial revolution*, so much urbanisation taking place, but the greatest change undoubtedly came in 1948 – with the introduction of the NHS. This country was then blessed with a *free* service (*for all except the elderly*) purportedly 'from cradle to grave'. Successive governments since then have failed to adequately maintain it financially and this *free* service has thus eventually 'broken down'. Either it must now be significantly changed *or private practice* needs to be restored! A solution and its outcome is beyond the horizons of this book.

From a medical viewpoint, Britain is beginning to look like a 'third world' country, and disease is now monitored by politicians rather than medically qualified individuals. What else can you thus expect?

How we miss the 'third world's *'extended family'*, and healthcare for the elderly especially – now that I (we) have joined the 90-year-olds – this both cares for and greatly respects the elderly. Britain's care of the ageing has also changed out of all recognition since the *nineteenth* century. As a medical practitioner, I have only scant sympathy towards the NHS's management and the British government of today in which the focus is largely on the *economy* while medicine and healthcare has been relegated to a minor rôle.[2]

It is clear therefore that medicine in Britain has changed immeasurably since I was a child; as the 'old fashioned' medical workforce has dwindled, former responsibilities of the *doctor* are subsiding and others, such as pharmacists and physiotherapists, are taking over. Greatest deterioration no doubt occurred following introduction of the NHS in 1948; the original aim of attending to everything from *'cradle to grave'* has certainly *not* been met however; although the cradle end of the spectrum is arguably the better, the right-hand is lying in ruins and has become a political rather than a medical matter! With increasing expenditure on medical practice, it seems unlikely that any country on this earth will be able to finance a *'free'* health service in the future.

Transition of a once great profession to the present 'shambles' (which for *political* reasons *must* survive) remains a sad reality. Personal experience in my lifetime confirms this! *There is no way I would pursue a medical career in this day and age.*

The outstanding need for integration of today's NHS with social care (*see also below*) has repeatedly been emphasised during the Covid-19 pandemic beginning in 2020. As Rachel Sylvester wrote in *The Times* newspaper, the '… starting point for a review is the quality of *social* care … the aim being to improve care given to the elderly … and they must reassure people that they will be looked after in old age without having to sell their home.' Should GPs visit care homes as apparently takes place for example in Manchester?

There is also currently a high 'turnover' in the care system; almost 80,000 healthcare workers leave their job annually! The pay is simply not in line with that of teachers and police officers. Social care is thus simply not attractive from a financial angle; according to Sylvester, 'you can earn more with less emotional strain working in a supermarket'. There needs urgently to be parity in the NHS until true integration takes place between health and social care … that must also give recognition to immigration because at present a perilously high proportion of healthcare workers comes from abroad. A tax rise for older workers – to pay for social care – is also being recommended. On the subject of loss of one's home in order to pay carers, this topic was addressed in subsequent *Times* correspondence, the answer being that an increased pension will only justify itself should you gain your health; those whose health *remains* good will have nothing to gain! Simply the reverse.[3]

Medicine and politics

In 1948 therefore, British medicine underwent a monumental change; this ancient discipline which for centuries had been administered by medically-trained people – often starting as apprentices – was taken over by politicians, usually without any form of medical training. Of all medical specialties, obstetrics has probably had the worst result since 1948! However, things have reached *crisis* point right across the board.

All initially went well, but the healthcare of the country was then comprehensively transferred and was now in the hands of a 'breed' of unscrupulous and dishonest inward-looking vote-hungry charlatans, most with absolutely no medical training or tuition. Of course the great profession thrived for a while (it had more finance than of late, and the voluntary hospitals which certainly had been in operation since 1123 (and possibly long before) in the time of Rahére – a monk), but what was to be the situation when Donald Trump (in the USA) or Boris Johnson (in Britain) came to power? The country was divided: more on the left-wing side were in favour of NHS survival (perhaps in a different form), while the right (led by the Conservative party – the more wealthy) were in favour of restoring *private* practice, although it would prove costly from a vote-winning angle! In fact, the situation was unsolved and it was difficult to discern a solution! . Strikes and disloyalty to such organisations as the *British Medical Association* (BMA) were on the horizon. The future seemed overall gloomy! Obviously, politicisation had brought a few advantages to medicine; if health had been as important to the politician as the economy, all would have been well, but it was way down the list.

What then can be salvaged from the wreckage? The younger generation (mostly born *after* inauguration of the NHS) know *no* other system of healthcare. The decaying NHS cannot be resuscitated without adequate funding; politicians have proved useless and the 'great profession' simply cannot afford to fund itself!

But present healthcare in Britain can't proceed like this; something must be done, but what? *Changes after 70 years have not been for the better in the long run. A fundamental component of H sapiens 'armoury' is now missing! Something must be done; politics is certainly not the answer.*[4]

Shortages of medical and nursing staff and serious ambulance delays in the NHS

There were numerous articles in British newspapers concerning reduction in medical and nursing staff – due to retirement (often premature) and also resignations – for dissatisfaction with service conditions etc, but *strikes* were unprecedented and certainly not even contemplated in my younger days; also standards are falling. There have also been records of serious ambulance delays – putting cardiac infarct patients' lives, for example, at serious risk During previous months numerous shortcomings in the NHS have been revealed, the *most* serious of which, to my mind, being those *not* involving direct medical matters, for example, staff shortages (*see above*) – but ambulance delays of many hours instead of a few minutes; it is these which account for many deaths.[5]

The British Medical Association (BMA)

The BMA has for long been known as the 'doctor's union'. It has to my knowledge previously been accepted as a *respectable* organisation; I am appalled that it has recently been mentioned in the context of 'industrial action' – another result of politicisation! Further evidence that medical standards are sinking is that diphtheria and poliomyelitis are both making a comeback (*see also above*). (It is true that in neither instance was the 'index case' in an indigenous person but nevertheless public health was involved.) These infections had previously been restricted to developing countries. Polio had been absent from these shores since introduction in the 1950s of satisfactory vaccines by Salk and Sabin.[6]

Striking doctors, nurses and others

Throughout my medical career, I had never previously heard of striking by medical practitioners. This is a form of protest *never* acceptable by members of the great profession and should not be accepted by a politically-run organisation. The mere mention of strikes never occurred in my earlier days after qualification. Its mention in daily newspapers is totally objectionable, and casts a gloomy eye on politically-run medicine, which has now hopefully had its run. Bring back the medical profession![7]

Social care

It was not until I had been personally taken to a care home at a cost of **£1,500 weekly** that I began to take an interest in social care! *On* taking office on 24 July 2019 the grossly dishonest British *Conservative* prime minister – a product of Eton College – promised to rapidly solve the long-standing *social care* problem. But when he was sacked on 6 September 2022, the situation had still not been advanced whatsoever!

The importance of *social care* and present inadequate funding is a 'stain on Britain', claimed *The Times* newspaper in July 2020. The architect of social care in David Cameron's proposed reform was Sir Andrew Dilnot, but sadly it was never implemented. As a corollary, Boris Johnson (*see above*), a subsequent Prime Minister, promised 'reforms to ensure that people no longer had to sell their homes to pay care bills.' Sir Andrew subsequently told MPs that the 'starting point [was] to *spend more* on social care.' He recommended a more generous testing threshold, and a cap on care costs, thus reducing the 'postcode lottery' for care services, and retaining disability benefits in a way that supported people's independence. This article received support from Lord

Warner, who in a letter indicated that the scheme would cost approximately '2 per cent of the present NHS budget', and is Part 1 of the 'Care Act 2014' which the government *could* activate and give (hard pressed) local authorities time and money to put administrative systems in place. Warner estimated that 'the end of 2021' *could* be the completion date.[8]

Medical research in 2022

Since I joined the 'great profession' I have become disappointed with the way in which it has relied almost entirely on 'established' (cast-iron and 'unbending') knowledge and how little is subject to modern research; two personal examples come to mind, *ie*: the view that *mefloquine* (an anti-malarial compound) is entirely without side-effects – when I know full well that in some people it has serious cerebral symptoms. Another example is *chronic fatigue syndrome* (CFS) which has numerous causes, whereas the *establishment 'knew'* (wrongly) that it was entirely psychiatric.[9]

Disease spectrum

During my medical career the spectrum of disease in Britain was largely that of the 'western' world – sucrose being a major causative factor in myocardial infarction, stroke, etc. while *infections* of all types (including tuberculosis) which were so frequent in the *nineteenth* century had fallen into the background; both medical personnel and sanatoria have for example adjusted accordingly. Now diseases of affluence are fading while *infectious* diseases are making a comeback, *eg* poliomyelitis and diphtheria (*see above*) are already becoming a curse of childhood previously thought of as 'third world' problems and now in the ascendance, much of it emanating from removed of 'tropical' forests. Epidemics and pandemics are thus likely to involve 'diseases' of the future. Covid-19 is one such, and as this slowly subsides, other viral diseases *eg* monkeypox are emerging; the WHO on 23 July 2022 issued an *International Health Emergency* warning with reference to this infection. With respect to infection abroad, Ghana has recently experienced three cases of Marburg disease (also a result of removal of West African forests, while Tanzania has recorded a case of rat-bite fever![10]

Present state of medicine in Britain and its future

We are living at a time of change. Even the *police* force which had its roots of course in the *Bow Street Runners,* requires significant alterations especially in its leadership. The same applies to medicine.

I have recently become amazed at certain remarks attributed to prominent MPs. Glowing credit has been given to Boris Johnson – a past Conservative prime minister – who is said to have *saved* the British population from the Covid-19 pandemic. In fact his presence at the helm during the recent pandemic most certainly does *not* justify this. Bring back the *medical profession* and sweep politicians aside! It is to be hoped that the great profession will soon be back in the hands of its rightful 'owners' rather than a group of power and vote-hungry politicians!

David Aaronovitch has written a valuable survey of the present state of the failing NHS, based on a report by Dr Axel Heitmueller on the future of that organisation. His *conclusions* were that 'it is [no longer] the glory of the world' and its 'central command' should be abolished. He is thus of the opinion that significant changes to basic infrastructure of the NHS are essential if it is to survive. In a reply in *The Times* correspondence column, having resigned from a partner in a GP practice he was reinstated under a GP retention scheme which it seems few knew about.[11]

The Times has rightly pointed out in a leading article that Britain anyway is no longer an attractive country for the young: wages are stagnant, taxes 'high, inflation rising, houses generally … unaffordable, and student debt is ballooning'; in fact young people have never before encountered such a gloomy scenario. What is to be done?

Owing to a variety of factors, general practice (GP) is suffering most; the London *Times* has predicted that by the year 2030, one in four GP posts will be unoccupied unless major changes are incorporated. **The basic and fundamental problem with healthcare in present-day Britain is that politics has displaced medicine since the NHS was created**. It is also true that we live in a 'different' world to that of 1948. Both Britain and the US, which has come to represent the 'West', are certainly not the same and both have lacked a good and effective leader! Even the mighty USA is not as 'cast iron' as one might suppose; the abortion and gun issues are both formidable and are dividing this 'massive' country in more ways than one. The long-lasting right to 'bear arms' in the second amendment of the constitution is a major issue which will not go away! And the recent reincarnation of the banning of abortion is obviously upsetting the female population throughout the land. So things are far less stable than one might suppose.

Conclusion

The future of the disaster-prone NHS seems *doomed*; it is likely in my judgement that healthcare in the hands of the Conservative party will be *privatised* anyway, and what will the poorer sections of the population do then? Now that Britain has stupidly withdrawn from the remainder of Europe and become even closer to the USA – 'Brexit' – in my view – I am very concerned about the future of medicine; many eminent *scientists* have already left Britain for mainland Europe and I fear that medicine might well go the same way. I am *not* in the business of predicting the *future*, but there is absolutely no doubt to my mind that the 1948 vision of *free* healthcare in Britain cannot rest with the NHS in its present form. Judging from the torrent of resignations and unfilled positions that feeling is widespread. *Britain simply must have a system of healthcare which is far superior to the present.*

Healthcare simply cannot remain in the hands of politicians; they have other matters to pursue and medicine (for which they are simply not trained) is *not* one of them!

The world and indeed Britain has changed beyond all recognition during my lifetime. There can be little doubt that general medical standards in the NHS are also sinking fast. Over the last few years, increasing numbers of patients have found the NHS not to meet their requirements. Can we *please* have the 'old fashioned' GP back?[12]

On 30 June 2023 the British media was focused on a set of proposed *solutions* to the NHS crisis. What were the politicians' 'inspired' changes to be made to a rapidly failing and politically-based healthcare service? The first and most vital reform was to solve monumental staff shortage(s); in order to attend to this, many more doctors and nurses will be trained and another five or so medical schools apparently opened! Furthermore, training-time for students of medicine will be reduced from five to four years; overall *thousands* of additional staff will thus be recruited; apprenticeships (which the medical profession had certainly seen before) will be reintroduced. I have serious doubts about shortening the medical course by twelve months; when I was a student, five years seemed far too short a time and several vital topics were thus 'crowded out'. This will inevitably lead to production of poorly-trained doctors! The present Prime Minister – Sunak – apparently welcomed these changes as 'the largest single expansion in NHS education in its history'.[13]

References and notes

1. P Morland. *A fortunate Woman: a country doctor's story.* London; Picador 2022: 235.
2. T Calver. 'It's no longer feasible to be a full-time GP': doctors' leader warns of working hours crisis'. *Sunday Times, Lond* 2022; 24 July: 1; Anonymous. No more task forces: the NHS crisis calls for tough decisions. *Ibid* 2022; 24 July: 22; Anonymous. No country for young people: stagnant wages, higher taxes, rising inflation, unaffordable houses and ballooning student debt. The young have never had it so tough. *Ibid* 2022; 1 July: 29; J Reynolds. Watchdog to investigate 40 new hospital pledge. *Ibid* 2022: 4 July: 4; E Hayward. Campaign to vaccinate children as the polio virus returns. *Times, Lond* 2022; 23 June: 1; E Hayward. Extra polio vaccine for 900,000 children to halt spread of virus. *Ibid* 2022; 11 August: 6; E Hayward. Race to trace 35,000 children at risk of polio. *Ibid* 2022; 24 June: 17; D M Davis. A little more vaccination: Elvis Presley and the race to beat polio. *Ibid* 2022; 26 June: 24; T Whipple, K Lay. Polio is back – but this could be its last stand rather than a revival. *Ibid* 2022; 25 June: 22; E Hayward. Polio survivors struggling with new symptoms decades later. *Ibid* 2022: 9 July: 38.
3. S Armstrong. Proof that our politicians really are a joke – at the Edinburgh Fringe. *Sunday Times, Lond* 2022; 14 August: 14; E Hayward. Burnout, bullying and sexism push NHS vacancies to 105,000. *Ibid* 2022; 25 July: 4; E Hayward. Pharmacies step in to help patients who can't see GPs. *Ibid* 2022; 30 December: 8.
4. M Barnier. *My Secret Brexit Diary: a glorious illusion.* USA: Polity Press 2021: 439; T Calver. Will we ever trust our politicians again: after the Brexit wars, 'partygate' and the legacy of the expenses scandal, a pressing task for whoever wins the keys to number 10 is to get a jaded public to believe a word they are saying. *Sunday Times, Lond* 2022; 28 August: 17; Anonymous. When voters lose faith in the NHS, Westminster must listen. *Ibid* 2022; 28 August: 20; K Lay. NHS staff and patients struggling. *Times, Lond* 2022; 22 June: 7; E Hayward. Patents pull own teeth in dentist crises. *Ibid* 2022; 22 June: 17; K Lay. Push to hire GPs overseas falls short. *Ibid* 2022; 25 June: 23; E Hayward. Doctors brand BMA sexist and racist. *Ibid* 2022; 29 June: 19; D Aaronovitch. NHS must take risks and innovate or die: if the health service ditches its central command, embraces data and accepts regional variation, it can yet prosper. *Ibid* 2022; 30 June: 27; K Gair.

BA online system refused to accept a female can be 'Dr.' *Ibid* 2022: 2 July: 11; A Smith. Two nations, divisible with anger and a sense of injustice for all. *Sunday Times, Lond* 2022: 3 July: 10; Anonymous. With leadership this poor, scandals can only get worse. *Ibid* 2022; 3 July: 32-3; A Seldon. Johnson taught us one valuable lesson: how *not* to be a prime minister: most holders of the highest office are forced out by scandal, coup or policy failure. The 85th PM was brought down by an unprecedented cocktail of all three. *Times, Lond* 2022: 9 July: 32-3; M Russell. Integrity in politics. *Ibid* 2022; 21 July: 28; D Haily. The dentist's chair. *Ibid;* 2022; 23 July: 28; N Colton. Are we ready to be radical – to fix the NHS – we are reluctant to look at how other countries fund their services. *Sunday Times, Lond* 2022: 21 August: 19; Anonymous. Care crisis: a further maternity scandal exposes the need for urgent reforms. *Times, Lond* 2022; 20 October: 33; E Hayward. More than half of maternity units now judged unsafe. *Ibid* 2022; 21 October: 14; S Lintern, B Spencer, T Calver, J Clover. Cancer waits rise to 55 days. *Sunday Times, Lond* 2022; 23 October: 7; B Chatworthy. Ambulance staff lead week of NHS strike votes. *Times, Lond* 2022; 24 October: 16; H Zeffman, C Smyth. Army to recue strike hit NHS. *Ibid* 2022; 28 November: 1; S Payne. *The Fall of Boris Johnson: The Full Story.* London Macmillan 2022: 275.

5. E Hayward. Surgeries struggle as 20,000 GPs plan to quit. *Times, Lond* 2022; 22 June: 1; K Lay. NHS staff and patients struggling. *Ibid* 2022; 22 June: 7; E Hayward. Patients pull own teeth in dentist crisis. *Ibid* 2022; 22 June: 17; E Hayward. Doctors demand 30% pay rise and warn of hospital pickets. *Ibid* 2022; 28 June: 2; E Hayward. One GP post in four to be empty by 2030. *Ibid* 2022; 30 June: 12; E Hayward. Doctor numbers drop to new low. *Ibid* 2022; 1 July: 18; J Brewerton. Retaining GPs. *Ibid* 2022; 2 July: 28; G Willoughby, A Lombardi, K Lay, E Hayward. Alarm over poor A&E care as 10% of patients return within a week. *Ibid* 2022; 4 July: 4; J W Tankel. NHS waiting lists. *Ibid* 2022; 9 July: 28; M Philips. NHS sacred cow must be put out of its misery; switching to a European model would stem the vast waste out of public money and raise standards. *Ibid* 2022; 26 July: 24. Anonymous. Full-time GPs at five year low. *Ibid* 2022; 29 July: 1; S Lintern, T Calver. Ambulance waits linked to thousands of deaths or life-changing injuries. *Ibid* 2022; 21 August: 4; Correspondence column. NHS shortfall. *Ibid* 2022; 12 September: 26; Correspondence column. Keeping NHS staff. *Ibid* 2022; 23 October: 28; E Hayward. Nurses leaving NHS in droves after 20% real-terms pay cut. *Ibid* 2022; 28 November: 14.

6. S Lintern. The war of the wards. BMA torn apart over pay and politics: as industrial action looms with doctors demanding 30% rises, the medical union is increasingly influenced by a left-wing alliance. *Sunday Times, Lond* 2022: 5 July: 4; C Wheeler, S Lintern, H Yorke. Manston failures led to migrant 'with diphtheria' being moved around UK. *Ibid* 2022; 27 November: 1,2; M Dathan. Migrant hotels sent diphtheria advice. *Times, Lond* 2022; 28 November: 9.
7. J Auchincloss. Striking doctors. *Ibid* 2022; 29 June: 3; A Cohn. Doctors' strike. *Ibid* 2022; 4 July: 24; C Smyth. Key lieutenant faces NHS strike and millions on waiting list. *Ibid* 2022; 6 July: 5; K Gair. Nurses balloted on strike action and winter walkout. *Ibid* 2022; 7 October 2; S Lintern. NHS consultants threaten to strike. *Sunday Times, Lond* 2022; 13 October: 11; Anonymous. All Out. *Times, Lond* 2022; 25 November: 39; Anonymous. Uncaring profession: for the first time, NHS consultants and junior doctors will this week strike on the same day. This reckless escalation makes them unworthy of public respect. *Ibid* 2023; 18 September: 31.
8. J Callery. Number waiting for social care soars 40% in a year. *Times, Lond* 2022; 14 May; R Blakeley. 'Brain drain' as scientists relocate to EU. *Ibid* 2022; 25 June: 2; R Sylvester. 'We've created our own brain drain … we don't attract the brightest and best'. *Ibid* 2022; 25 June; Anonymous. Science in limbo: The EU stand-off over Northern Ireland threatens vital research in Britain. *Ibid* 2022; 25 June: 29.
9. A M Ramsay. Outbreak at the Royal Free. *Lancet* 1955 2: 391; G C Cook. Melfoquine toxicity should limit treatment. *Br med J* 1995 311: 190-1; D Strain. Action plan for ME. *Ibid* 2022 13 May: 30; S T Highgate. New stance on ME. *Ibid* 2022 20 May: 30; S O'Neil. Hunt begins work for genes to unlock mystery of ME. *Ibid* 2022 12 September: 26; G Sandeman. ME patient told 'you're making it up'. *Ibid* 2022; 28 September: 12.
10. J Hunt. *Zero: eliminating unnecessary deaths in a post-pandemic NHS*. London Swift Press 2022: 303; K Lay. Six children dead from Strep A after infection cases quadruple. *Times, Lond* 2022; 3 December: 6; K Lay. Act quickly on Strep A infection to avoid more child deaths, GPs urged. *Ibid* 2022; 5 December: 6; K Lay, C Wace. Take children with Strep A straight to A&E, says peer. *Ibid* 2022; 6 December: 11; S Lintern. Desperate parents search for Strep A medicine as prices soar. *Sunday Times, Lond* 2022; 11 December: 1; A Ellison. Drug suppliers warned over steep rise in cost of Strep A antibiotics. *Times, Lond* 2022; 13 December: 8; E Hayward. Strep A kills more children as fever cases hit new high. *Ibid* 2022: 23 December: 3.

11. B Spencer, R Lavin, J Coff. Ireland charges £50 to see a GP. Could it be the bitter pill the NHS needs? *Sunday Times, Lond* 2022; 27 November: 13.
12. S Murray. *The future of Medicine* London Penguin Books 1942: 126; E Duncan. NHS must start saying 'no' if it wants to survive: too many high-risk patients are having surgery with poor outcomes for both them and society. *Ibid* 2022; 29 July: 29; K Lay, *et al*. Patients turn to private GPs. *Times, Lond* 2022 28 May: 11; Anonymous. Spent Force: special measures for the metropolitan police are long overdue. But only a wholesale change of leadership can save the organisation now. *Ibid* 2022; 30 June: 31; G Baker. Angry, divided mistrustful: is this how America ends? *Times, Lond* 2022; 2 July: 32-3; K Lay. NHS dying of Covid, say journal chiefs. *Ibid* 2022; 19 July 16; J Flanagan. Three die from illness linked to rats and bats. *Ibid* 2022; 19 July: 30; B Lagan. Even lonely Pitcairn can't escape the spread of Covid. *Ibid* 2022; 19 July: 30; E Hayward. The medic taking scalpel to NHS sexism. *Ibid* 2022; 23 July: 14; Correspondence column. Sacred cow of NHS. *Ibid* 2022; 27 July: 28; A Nachlappan. 100,000 drop out of work suffering from long Covid. *Ibid* 2022; 27 July: 16; Correspondence column. How to treat our struggling health service. *Ibid* 29 July: 28; R Colville. They say Britain's broken but the good news is we're in a state of transition, not collapse. *Ibid* 2022; 14 August: 24. Anonymous. Cancel Culture; the Queen's funeral ought not to be cause for the NHS to deny patient care. *Ibid* 2022; 18 September: 31.
13. K Lay, C Smyth. Blueprint to boost NHS workforce by 300,000: plan will speed up trainees' route to wards. *Times, Lond* 2023; 30 June: 1, 2.

APPENDIX: Nutritional research in southern Africa:

My 'academic' contributions in Zambia

When I arrived in Lusaka to take up my new position in late 1969 – Professor of (academic) Medicine in the capital city of Zambia (formerly Northern Rhodesia) – independence from colonial rule was still being celebrated. Kenneth Kaunda ([1924-2021]) was president and future course of country and university were still being developed. The totally unacceptable practice of *apartheid* remained in operation in nearby South Africa.

There are two 'subsections' of *Homo sapiens*: those with an 'enquiring mind' constantly attempting to solve problems, and others who are content with the *status quo*. My basic instinct was with the former and I was delighted therefore to have been appointed to (Dame) Sheila Sherlock (1918-2001)'s department where I learned a great deal about *academic* medicine. Historically, progress has depended almost entirely on 'original thinkers' such as William Harvey (1576-1657) for *progress* in medicine. In common with teaching, *clinical research* is a topic which divided minds of many during this era, now half a century ago.*[6] Some favoured medical practice and research on an *international* basis, and others 'down-to-earth' medicine which was strictly 'tailored' to the needs of the country under consideration (Zambia, or later Papua New Guinea [PNG]). The latter subscribers were critical of my programme(s) which they considered too 'high-powered' for a developing country! This is a view taken

---

6 * I have always believed that students must be able to physically examine a patient; British clinical medicine is unlike that practised in the USA– where investigations always come first.

by most 'Christian missionaries' and championed by the late George Nelson, a member of the UK's *Tropical Medicine Research Board* which represented Britain's *Medical Research Council* (MRC) when on a visit of inspection in 1973. I later discovered that it was also a view of a colleague – Zumla at *University College Hospital, London.*

I had by 1969, been employed by *Makerere University College*, Kampala, Uganda for two years where I had imbibed first-hand knowledge of a developing country's outstanding post-colonial agenda which certainly had an *international* ring! It was my ambition and intention to make the new *Department of Medicine* in Zambia equal to *Mulago Hospital* in Uganda which had been responsible for several major original research contributions – including geographical distribution of the lymphoma named after Denis Burkitt (1911- 93) FRCS, FRS. This was my target! I had also personally already pioneered a great deal of work on small-intestinal structure and function in Uganda, including the *lactase* enzyme, summarised in a book – *The Milk Enzyme* (*see below*).

Soon after arrival in Lusaka, I had decided to investigate *small-intestinal absorption* of the dietary components of most rural Zambians, and in particular the influence of *infections* (acute and chronic) on that process. Much of my work involved use of a double-lumen tube intubation technique, a *non-invasive* method with which I had become familiar at the *Royal Free Hospital* in London. My mentor throughout was Tony (later Sir Anthony) Dawson, then a physician at St Bartholomew's Hospital, London and later also physician to HM Queen Elizabeth II (1926-2022). Enrolment of suitable volunteers was to a large extent left to my *clinical assistant* – a Zambian African by the name of James Tembo (*see below*). Most investigations are recorded in the following pages. Early work was performed in the old hospital (*Lusaka Central Hospital*) in unsophisticated surroundings, and later ones at the *new University Teaching Hospital* (UTH). In Lusaka and also Kampala, Riyadh and Port Moresby, I personally carried out *all* biochemical determinations. Although we employed a technician in the department of medicine in Zambia, he dealt only with routine haematology etc, all *research* determinations being done by myself, often *out of hours,* and to my satisfaction they reached the level of excellence which one would accept as part of a *research project*.

A somewhat confused forecast of my future research in Zambia was published in a local newspaper, *The Times of Zambia*. In September 1970 (*ie* soon after my 'reign' in Zambia had begun) this newspaper announced:

the *Lions Club* is to finance a K [Kina] 20,000 nutrition research project to be carried out shortly at the [UTH], *Lusaka*. The … research aims at establishing that malnutrition in Zambia and other developing countries may be practically due to … difficulty in digestion of protein, and also to eating too much food with [a] high carbohydrate [and] low protein content. The K20,000 will be used for buying apparatus … used to analyse the protein content of diets and the way in which protein is absorbed from the intestine. Approaches to order a machine from England or Australia have already been made by the Lions Club. The apparatus will be especially manufactured for the purpose.

The man carrying out the research is Professor Gordon Cook of the *University of Zambia*. Professor Cook, who has worked on problems of nutrition and absorption for more than five years, said his main interest in the investigations will be the absorption of carbohydrate and protein foods from the intestines. He said it has been shown in many parts of Africa that absorption of these substances takes place much more slowly in Africans than in Europeans and Americans, whose food is usually rich in protein. … Professor Cook has already proved that when someone eats a meal with a very high content of carbohydrate [and] little protein, the carbohydrates slow … absorption of the protein. He is carrying out further work on this problem.

'Malnutrition here and in other developing counties has always been solely associated with lack of food but I feel this impairment in absorption must [also] have something to do with it, and that is what I am working on,' Professor Cook said. As [an associated] theme, [he] is also interested in the cause of heart attacks, which are very common in Europeans and Americans [but to date do *not*] occur in Africans. This might be due to [a] difference in diet but could … be associated with differences in absorption, he said. Professor Cook, 38, was trained at *London University* where he completed his MD, BSc and MRCP [sic] degrees. He qualified in [1957]. Since then he has worked on and off in several London hospitals. He served as an army medical specialist in Nigeria in 1961-1962. Before coming to Zambia last year, he taught (and carried out research) at *Makerere University College* in Uganda.[1]

That proposed grant failed to materialise and I suspected at the time that the Lion's Club had to some extent or other been influenced by the 'missionary element' (*see above*) and that this research was at that time considered too sophisticated and 'high powered' for Zambia! Dawson's colleagues at *St Bartholomew's* generously shared their thoughts and ideas with me.

To summarise my 1969-70 position:

- One was dealing with an unsophisticated (and mostly uneducated) population, who incorrectly anticipated from the outset that the *new* department would be oriented simply and *entirely* around *cure of the individual*, and that other functions of an *academic* department, *ie* both teaching medical students and nurses, and *research*, were simply unnecessary, and furthermore harmful to a sick patient. Apartheid was firmly implanted in South Africa, and the *white* man was at that time extremely unpopular.

- *clinical research* was *certainly* considered *not* to be a priority, and

- another difficulty was that most, possibly all, of my staff had previously *not* set foot in an *internationally-acceptable academic Department of Medicine*: *clinical* research was thus an entirely new and novel pursuit to them.

In my view excellent *clinical* research was essential to every worthwhile department of medicine in both the developed and developing world. First-class research published in appropriate journals is essential to establishing the department as a centre of *international* excellence. A new department *not* backed by sound research will never succeed in a *world* setting! My *clinical* research in *Lusaka* can be summarised under five headings (*see below*). But before embarking on a summary of results, I shall briefly refer to the non-invasive perfusion-system which I evaluated with assistance of a surgical colleague – Richard Carruthers FRCS.

It is of course impossible to predict the outcome of scientific research – one could be heading down a strictly 'blind alley'. My personal research in Lusaka was retrospectively summarised in an article in the journal *Gut* in 1974:[2]

- *adult hypolactasia* (on which I had previously worked in Uganda),

- effect of *systemic infection* and *malnutrition* on *carbohydrate, amino-acid* and *di-peptide* absorption,

- *amino-acid* absorption,

- *monosaccharide* absorption, and

- *mechanisms* involved in intestinal absorption.

I – Validation of the small-intestinal perfusion technique and site of maximum intestinal absorption

In order to quantify effect of intestinal *'concertinaing'* and its influence on absorption area, *six* people undergoing an *elective* abdominal laparotomy were studied:

> Marked 'concertinaing' (or gathering) of small-intestine *proximal* to the mercury weight at the distal end of the tube was confirmed at laparotomy in each person. The ratio between mean intestinal-length from weight to ligament of Treitz – after removal of the tube to that with the tube *in situ* – was 3.0 (2.5-3cm). Mean total jejuno-ileal length was 421 (320-521) cm. In *five* of the *six* people, distal end of the tube was over 50% of distance between Treitz and ileo-caecal valve, although only 100-120 (mean 108) cm distant from incisor teeth.

> Segmental perfusion studies of human jejunum therefore involved a longer length of small-intestine (a factor of approximately three) than generally assumed. Such studies assess absorption *rate* over a significant proportion of small-intestine and are thus *not* confined to a *short* segment of *proximal* jejunum; the nutritional significance of studies in which amino-acids, peptides, and carbohydrates were evaluated is thus *increased*. Studies designed to measure absorption-*rate* from the ileum should be treated with caution since part or all of the perfused segment might be *distal* to the ileo-caecal valve.[3]

Substances undergoing investigation were *always* perfused in 'random' order and thus the 'concertinaing' effect was identical with every perfusion.

Because this procedure measures *rate* and not *overall absorption*, I also carried out an investigation, the result of which was perhaps unexpected but nevertheless also validated findings of investigations using the double-lumen tube technique.

It was also important to identify the precise area of small-intestine at which *maximal* absorption occurs.

Glucose given orally was previously shown to be absorbed largely in *first* part of small-intestine. However, there are only limited data on whether or not absorption can also take place in *distal* small-intestine. Impairment of glucose absorption in presence of *systemic* bacterial infection, and mutual inhibition between glucose and glycine absorption in *proximal* jejunum might both be important in human nutrition (*see below*); it is important to know therefore whether glucose absorption is possible in *distal* jejunum. Glucose infused into *proximal* jejunum is shown to produce a greater rise in plasma insulin than when administered intravenously; blood glucose and insulin responses to glucose at various sites of *proximal* jejunum were also compared with those during *intravenous* infusion given at the same rate in *six* relatively normal Zambian Africans.

This investigation clearly indicates therefore that in Africans glucose absorption can take place over a limited section of *proximal* small-intestine and is possible at 50 cm (or more) past Treitz. Obviously this observation is potentially important nutritionally.[4]

The findings of these two investigations were of enormous confirmatory significance in interpretation of subsequent studies using the double-lumen tube technique in relevance to human nutrition, *eg* importance of *proximal* small-intestinal absorption in overall practical nutritional requirement of rural Zambians and others in 'third-world' countries.

Solutes chosen for perfusion studies were:

Lactose – disulpharide
Glucose – monosaccharide
Acyl-glycine   )
)
L Histidine   ) amino acids
)
Methionine   )

Glycylglycine – di-peptide

II – Adult Hypolactasia (low jejunal lactase concentration) in adult-life

The intestinal *lactase* saga began around 1960; prior to that it was assumed that *all adults* world-over designated *Homo sapiens* possess an abundance of *lactase* at the enterocytic brush-border. However, my research in Uganda (summarised in *The Milk Enzyme – see below*) indicated that while most members of *H sapiens* in northern Europe retain that enzyme into *adult* life (PL), that is *not* so in the vast majority of African descent. It was later demonstrated that this situation applied to the majority of the world's human population and possesses a *genetic* basis; there is now *overwhelming evidence* that adult hypolactasia is *not* an acquired condition – due to either lack of dietary *lactose* or perhaps another factor, but is the *normal* state for all adult mammals, except most northern Europeans, their descendants and the Hamitic people of northern Africa or the middle-east, who have consumed milk and/or milk products for probably thousands of years. In a Finnish study evidence indicates that the condition is inherited by a *single recessive autosomal gene*.

It is suggested that high *lactase* concentration in most adult northern Europeans has resulted from a selective advantage associated with increased calcium absorption in population groups which have been exposed for centuries to low ultraviolet radiation and vitamin D intake. However, that observation does not explain the high incidence of *lactase persistence* (PL) in Hamitic tribes of east Africa. Lactose tolerance may however merely be associated with an unspecific nutritional advantage of milk which has been consumed by man in adult-life for perhaps only 4000 to 6000 years.[5]

In order to determine the *lactase* situation in *adult* Zambian Africans, I therefore analysed, with assistance of collaborators in Sweden, the situation in Lusaka. Almost 100% have *hypolactasia* as shown by low *lactase* concentration in jejunal biopsies (*see below*). In an extension of this investigation and by using the double-lumen tube method (*see above*), I also demonstrated that that enzyme status reflects the physiological situation, *ie* lactose was extremely poorly absorbed from the jejunum, and thus influenced net water movement *towards* the small-intestinal lumen; in that study, lactose solutions of 50, 125 and 250 mM were used. Milk (which of course contains lactose) given orally is associated with small-intestinal fluid transfer (exudation) and in a high percentage of adults, initiates diarrhoea. There is also evidence from that study that a small amount of lactose enters the enterocyte intact.

Kinetic curves for lactose absorption were constructed as part of my *clinical* research in *six* Zambian African adults. Since glucose absorption from maltose (100 mM) occurs at a significantly greater rate than from glucose (200 mM) in Zambian African adults, it is possible that that observation can be partly explained by absorption of some of intact disaccharide.[6]

Before travelling to Zambia (in late 1969) I had also worked in Nigeria (1961-2) and Uganda (1965-7). In the latter country I carried out a great deal of research into *hypolactasia* in Ugandan Africans. I felt it almost a duty therefore to ascertain the *lactase*-status of indigenous adults in Zambia; two investigations were designed with this in mind. Apart from genetic significance, I considered it an important cause of infant and childhood malnutrition (*marasmus*). These investigations were thus centred on incidence of the enzyme's polymorphism, the second of which utilised the double-lumen system of small-intestinal perfusion to study absorption kinetics *in vivo*.

Some African tribes, *ie* those with north African or middle-eastern ancestry, have a *lactase* concentration in *adult*-life similar to that of most Europeans.[7] A summary of the *first* investigation on *lactase* carried out with the Swedish group was:

> Activities of brush-border *lactase*, lysosomal acid ß-galactosidase and cytoplasmic hetero-ß-galactosidase were measured in jejunal-biopsies from 26 Zambian Africans; all had *adult hypolactasia*. Low activity of brush-border *lactase* amounted to 5 to 90 (mean 62)% of total *lactase* activity at *p*H 6.0. Acid ß-galactosidase and hetero-ß-galactosidase activities however were *not* decreased. Oral lactose 'tolerance' tests were 'abnormal' in 25, and 21 had gastrointestinal symptoms. There was a significant correlation between *brush-border lactase* activity and maximum blood glucose rise following oral lactose, indicating that low concentration of this enzyme in Zambian Africans is adequate for hydrolysis of a significant fraction of oral lactose.

The *second* investigation can be summarised as follows:

> Using the double-lumen tube perfusion system (*see above*), solutions of lactose (50, 125 and 250 mmol/l) were introduced into upper jejunum of *six* Zambian Africans. By reference to the non-absorbable marker, polyethylene glycol (mol. wt 4000), rates of lactose absorption from each solution was calculated for a 30 cm jejunal segment. In three total *lactase* activity in jejunal mucosa, brush-border *lactase* and other disaccharidase activities were estimated. Jejunal total and brush-border *lactase* activities were all low, while jejunal morphology was normal for Africans. All suffered abdominal colic and diarrhoea during and following the lactose perfusions. Kinetic curves for lactose were shallow, and with all perfused solutions there was net movement of water towards the jejunal lumen. Limited numbers and narrow range of enzyme activity did *not* permit significant correlation between lactose absorption-rate and activity. In Zambian Africans with *adult hypolactasia*, jejunal mucosa absorbs only a very small proportion of perfused lactose.

It is therefore clear that the vast majority of Zambian Africans have *hypolactasia* in adult life (as predicted) and are thus 'normal' in the context of

Nutritional significance of hypolactasia

Absence of brush-border *lactase* in adult life is unlikely to be associated with significant ill-health; intolerance to lactose (in milk) is nevertheless common in most adult Africans and Asians. Following seven to 10 days of regular (daily) milk intake (at 0.5 to 1 litre) however, a marked degree of tolerance can be acquired despite the fact that brush-border *lactase* concentration is *not* altered; the mechanism of that response is so far unknown. Clearly therefore, adult Zambians who are unwell (due to another cause) should *not* be given oral milk.

In Zambian African babies and infants on the other hand a high incidence of non-infective diarrhoea has been demonstrated and this readily responds to discontinuance of milk; it seems likely that that is frequently due to an early fall in jejunal *lactase* to a low adult concentration. How frequently milk *intolerance* is causally related to nutritional *marasmus* (energy malnutrition) is however to date unknown.[8]

III – Effect of systemic infection and malnutrition on absorption

Effect of systemic infection and malnutrition on xylose, glucose, glycine and glycylglycine absorption

Most of Zambia's population subsists on a staple diet – maize (sweetcorn) which consists of *maltose* combined with a limited amount of protein in the form of various amino-acids (tryptophan and lysine being largely omitted) together with several peptides. My first inclination on being in Zambia was to carry out research on effect(s) of *systemic infection* (common in that environment) on *glucose* (major constituent of maltose), *amino-acid* and *peptide* absorption. Evidence indicated that most glucose, glycine and glycylglycine absorption takes place in *proximal* small-intestine, work on glucose *absorption* site indicating that most absorption occurs in *proximal* rather than *distal* jejunum (*see above*).

The first firm indication that *systemic infection* (*acute* and *chronic*) exerts a significant effect on absorption came from Zambians who volunteered for D-xylose absorption tests.

Absorption of D-xylose is frequently mildly impaired in normal Africans, this being shown to apply to others in tropical countries. Although correlation with severity of histological abnormality of jejunal mucosa has been demonstrated, that has *not* been confirmed in another investigation. In Ugandan Africans, D-xylose absorption is frequently impaired in presence of normal mucosa. In a group of Zambian African patients, mean D-xylose (25gm) excretion was significantly lower in those with acute and chronic *infections*.[9]

This led to a study involving *glucose* absorption in presence of *systemic infection*:

> Using the double-lumen perfusion system (*see above*), absorption of *glucose* from 56, 139 and 278 mM solutions was compared in groups with *systemic infection* and controls, infections consisting of *acute* (lobar pneumonia) or *chronic* (respiratory tuberculosis) illnesses; no patient in this study had either malnutrition or gastrointestinal disease. Those with infections had a statistically significant reduction in glucose absorption-*rate*. D-xylose and glucose almost certainly share an identical transfer mechanism.[10]

Absorption-*rate* of glycine from 100, 150, and 250 mM solutions was however significantly raised in those with *infection* (see below) suggesting that this indicated an adaptive conservation of amino-acid in presence of a high catabolic rate – associated with *infection*.[11]

Regarding the di-peptide *glycylglycine* – which seems to utilise a separate transfer mechanism to that of glycine (see below) – absorption-rate from a 50 mM solution was *not* absorbed differently in those with *infections* (see below). This confirms evidence that the di-peptide pathway is less affected by *infection* than that of an amino-acid.[12]

The *conclusion* from these studies was therefore that most indigenous people in a developing country such as Zambia suffering from either an *acute* or *chronic* bacterial infection lose countless calories from the monosaccharide *glucose* during periods of infection (acute or chronic), while the mechanism for amino-acid absorption becomes increasingly efficient; that for di-peptides is unaltered. An 'adaptive' mechanism for amino-acids *during* an acute or chronic infection would *not* though be possible in people (eg most Zambians) subsisting on a *marginal* amino-acid source! These initial studies were strongly supported by others on γ-globulin and IgG concentrations and on their relationship to absorption of other dietary constituents (*see below*).[13]

Raised γ-globulin-concentration in serum of Zambian Africans usually results from bacterial and parasitic infection – most importantly malaria. Significant *inverse* correlations between globulin and IgG concentrations and *glucose* absorption from *proximal* jejunum were demonstrated. These are consistent with previous conclusions, and must emphasise the massive influence of *systemic infection* on absorption-rate. Also in line with previous results is the fact that correlation between elevated serum globulin and glycylglycine absorption-rate was *not* significant. Thus there seemed to be a clear correlation between absorption-rate and absorption of all substances studied.

Serum Globulin and Albumin Concentration

As a corollary to these observations on an *overt* systemic infection, the following represents likely implications of a *covert* systemic infection on absorption and subsequent disease. A significant *inverse* association was demonstrated in Zambian Africans *without* clinical evidence of an infection (or gastrointestinal disease) between glucose absorption-rate (from a 200 mM solution) from *proximal* jejunum, and serum total and ɣ-globulin concentration. Raised serum ɣ-globulin concentration in most Africans are probably largely due to bacterial and parasitic disease, most importantly intestinal parasites and malaria. A further study has shown that impaired glucose absorption-rate is inversely related to serum IgG concentration but *not* significantly to IgM, IgA, or IgD. It therefore seems likely that impairment of glucose absorption-rate associated with *systemic infection* is directly related to raised serum ɣ-globulin, and more specifically to elevated serum IgG concentration. Whether high ɣ-globulin concentration is associated with abnormal membrane transfer at other sites has *not* been determined. For *glycine*, a significant positive relationship between jejunal absorption-rate (from a 100 mM solution) and serum total and ɣ-globulin concentration was demonstrated; that adds to demonstration of *increased* glycine absorption-rate in those with an *acute systemic infection*. A significant association was *not* however demonstrated between serum globulin concentration and glycine absorption-rate from a 50 mM glycylglycine solution (*see above*).

In an investigation in Lagos, Nigeria it has been suggested, on limited evidence, that subclinical malabsorption in Nigerians is directly associated with low serum *albumin* concentration. In Zambian Africans without *clinical* evidence of infection or gastrointestinal disease no significant association between absorption-rate of glucose, glycine, glycylglycine and serum *albumin* concentration were demonstrated.[14]

I had at this point become fascinated by potential importance of *systemic* infection on absorption of other dietary substances. Owing to absence of suitable facilities in Lusaka, the following investigation had to await my return to the

UK. Having established a significant effect on several nutritional substances, albeit at relatively high concentration, on intestinal absorption-rate it therefore seemed of interest to assess effect of systemic infection on absorption-rate of *folic acid*. In a limited study, an overwhelming reduction on folic acid (pteroylglutamic acid) absorption was demonstrated; should this apply to *dietary* folic acid, it might be important in reduction in *systemic* infection.[15]

Nutritional significance

Having obtained this information, indicating a significant effect of *systemic* infection on absorption-rate of various chemical (and dietary) constituents, it is clearly important to apply this to other dietary factors also. At least one essential ingredient is frequently present at a marginal concentration in the diet of a vast proportion of the world's human population; since demonstration in the early 1930s by Dr Cecily Williams (1893-1992) (who I had had the pleasure of meeting in Lusaka in 1972) that kwashiorkor is the result of a low protein intake – followed by diminished *serum* protein concentration, malnutrition in tropical countries has usually been considered *entirely* of dietary origin(*see below*). That viewpoint has since dominated the scene, while other factors especially *malabsorption* of various dietary constituents are in fact also important in pathogenesis. In developing countries 'energy' and protein are often present at low concentration on an average diet. For example, the majority of Zambian Africans survive on a carbohydrate diet which contains only marginally adequate amounts of protein, the staple diet in most regions of the country being *nshima*, a 'porridge' prepared from ground maize (or millet). Although childhood malnutrition is common, *adults* are moderately well nourished compared with those in numerous other tropical locations.

In most studies cited, concentration of mono- and disaccharides, amino-acids and di-peptides in the perfusing fluid were probably higher than present *in vivo* at the luminal surface of the enterocyte in the *proximal* jejunum, although there are few existent data to support that. Whether or not absorption-rate in *proximal* jejunum bears a significant relationship to *total* absorption of dietary protein and carbohydrate is not overwhelmingly clear (*see above*). A significant correlation has been demonstrated between absorption-rate of glucose from *proximal* jejunum, and weight of D-xylose excreted after a 25g oral load. Similarly, a significant correlation has been demonstrated between D-xylose absorption (from a jejunal segment) and excretion after an oral load; there are only limited data available on amount of those solutes which can be absorbed overall if not *proximally*. Glucose is clearly rapidly absorbed from *proximal* jejunum of Zambian Africans (*see above*), while there is evidence of limited absorption in *distal* small-intestine. Evidence exists that the amino-acid L-methionine (*see below*) is absorbed more rapidly from *proximal* than *distal* small-intestine of *H sapiens*; however, glycine seems well absorbed in *distal* small-intestine.

Most indigenous people in a tropical country live largely on carbohydrate in some form or other. It seems probable therefore that my observations have important nutritional significance. In a highly developed community – such as Britain – increased amino-acid absorption-rate is possible during an *acute* infection and that carries an additional energy requirement; however, in an African or Asian community low dietary amino-acid availability would preclude an adaptive response. Energy intake from carbohydrate would be reduced *during* an infection due to impaired glucose absorption-rate. Systemic infection would as a result be related to production of malnutrition by way of impaired absorption, in Uganda a close seasonal association being demonstrated between a systemic bacterial and/or viral infection, as well as *acute* gastrointestinal infection, and time of onset of *kwashiorkor*. Although much of that association is probably mediated by high catabolic rate associated with systemic infection, *reduced absorption might also be important.* Since *rate* of *glycylglycine* absorption is *not* increased in people with a bacterial infection, it seems possible that protein supplements in the form of amino-acids rather than peptides given to patients with an infection will be more effective even though in normal circumstances the former are absorbed more slowly than the latter.

Effect of malnutrition on absorption-rates of glucose, glycine and glycylglycine

In order to extend observations on intestinal absorption in those with malnutrition in Zambia, the following investigation was undertaken:

> Absorption rate of glucose (from a 200 mM solution), glycine (100 mM solution), and glycylglycine (50 mM) were estimated in *six* Zambian African adults with *clinical* malnutrition. The double-lumen tube technique was used to determine absorption-rate from a 30 cm jejunal segment *in vivo*. Mean serum albumin concentration was 24 (14-43) g/l. Absorption rate was compared with that of Zambian Africans (controls) previously studied, without *clinical* evidence of malnutrition, systemic infection or gastrointestinal disease. Mean glucose, glycine and glycylglycine absorption-rate in malnourished people were *not* significantly different from controls.

Mean net water absorption-rate from glucose solution was similar in malnourished volunteers and controls during glycine and glycylglycine perfusions, mean net absorption-rate being significantly lower in the malnourished. Mean net water transfer was towards the jejunal lumen during glycine perfusion in the malnourished. One volunteer with pellagra had abnormal D-xylose excretion after a 25g oral load; all other tests were normal.

It seems probable therefore that *malnutrition* must be *very* severe – with jejunal mucosal abnormality – before absorption-rate of glucose, glycine and glycylglycine are significantly altered. This study does *not* therefore support the view that *subclinical* malnutrition is important in production of overt malabsorption of dietary components in Zambian Africans. Systemic bacterial infection and raised serum ɣ-globulin and immunoglobulin IgG concentration seem more likely than *subclinical malnutrition* to be relevant in context of absorption, in genesis of *overt* malnutrition.[16]

IV – Amino-acid absorption

Other amino-acids and monosaccharides were introduced into the perfusion fluid largely in order to assess interaction. Absorption-rate of L-methionine from a 100 mM solution was impaired by glucose (150 mM) in the perfusion fluid in *six*, but two others showed an *increase*, overall effect of glucose on *L-methionine* absorption-rate *not* being significant. The mechanism responsible for a mutually inhibitive effect of glucose and galactose on glycine absorption-rate from jejunum is unknown, but could be related to excessive demands on a common energy supply in jejunal mucosa or an allosteric interaction at brush-border surface; whether this observation has a practical value in human nutrition is unknown, and more data are required concerning concentration of monosaccharides, amino-acids and peptides presented to the luminal enterocyte *in vivo*. It seems reasonable to suppose that any degree of impairment in amino-acid absorption in those living on a high carbohydrate diet with a marginally adequate amount of amino-acid *must* assume importance.

V – Monosaccharide absorption and influence of other 'food ingredients'

'Flat' Oral Glucose Tolerance curve and Impaired D-xylose excretion in Zambian Africans

A 'flat' blood-glucose curve after oral glucose (50 or 100g) and low excretion of D-xylose following a 25g oral load are relatively common in Africans – living in Africa – although there is frequently no obvious *clinical* evidence of disease (Cook, G C, *personal observation*). It now seems extremely unlikely that jejunal mucosal morphology of Africans living in Africa – which only differs mildly from English people in England – is responsible for such abnormalities, even though jejunal surface area is undoubtedly compromised compared with Europeans living in a temperate country, the mucosa usually consisting of broad, leaf-shaped villi with occasional ridges and only rarely finger-shaped ones. In some Zambian Africans with jejunal morphology characteristic of Africans, glucose absorption-rate and D-xylose excretion are identical to results obtained in Europeans in the United Kingdom. Although absorption-rate used in glucose absorption studies presently cited was lower than in a study on English subjects in England, mean kinetic curve in Zambian Africans *without* infection is flatter. Many Africans have a high serum γ-globulin, usually due to elevated serum IgG. That has been associated with impaired glucose and D-xylose absorption. It seems likely, therefore, that frequent occurrence of a 'flat' oral glucose 'tolerance' curve and an abnormal D-xylose test (in Zambian Africans) is associated with that observation.[17]

VI – *Absorptive mechanisms*

Although my studies had clear objectives in view, they also inadvertently threw important light on *intestinal absorption mechanisms*. Initial studies demonstrated *competition* between monosaccharides and amino-acids. Incorporating both glucose and galactose (200 mM), significant interference with glycine (100 mM) absorption-rate was also demonstrated.

An increase amounting to about 30% – of a diet containing marginal amino-acid concentration would amount to overwhelming nutritional significance. However, at lower concentration, inhibition was less, and in some cases failed to reach statistical significance. The fact that *glycylglycine, a di-peptide,* absorption-rate was unaltered in presence of infection was unexpected. But a significant *decline* in *glucose* absorption-rate indicates that energy (calorie) supplies – derived from food – would also be reduced by up to 30% (confirmed by serum γ-globulin and IgG concentrations) was also unexpected and shown to be a major precipitating factor in protein-energy malnutrition, including *kwashiorkor* (*see above*).

Remaining studies (primarily physiological) were aimed at assessment of (i) effect of glycine (an amino-acid) on glycylglycine (a di-peptide) absorption-rate, (ii) glycine and another amino-acid on glucose and galactose absorption-rates, and (iii) glucose and maltose absorption-rate. All patients from now were free of *systemic* infection.

Comparison of absorption-rate of glycine and glycylglycine alone and combined with glucose

Using the perfusion system (*see* above) rates of glycine, glycylglycine, and glycylglycine + glucose absorption were studied in a group of relatively normal Zambian Africans *in vivo*. To construct a kinetic curve for glycine absorption, *four* were given consecutive perfusions containing 50, 100 and 150 mM. *Six* others had consecutive perfusions of (i) 100 mM-glycine and (ii) 50mM-glycylglycine solution; *five* had a higher absorption-rate of glycine from glycylglycine. When data from a further *six* volunteers in another study were included, mean glycine absorption-rate was significantly faster from glycylglycine than glycine solution. A further *six* had consecutive perfusions of (i) 50 mM-glycylglycine, (ii) 50 mM-glycylglycine + 200 mM-glucose, and (iii) 200 mM-glucose. Absorption-rate of glycine from glycylglycine was lower in *all* volunteers when glucose was present in perfusing fluid; this difference was *not* significant.

Comparison of glycine and glycylglycine absorption-rates

Absorption of glycine and glycylglycine were compared *in vivo* when those compounds were given alone or together to *six* Zambian Africans who lacked *clinical* evidence of both malnutrition and gastro-intestinal disease. Solutions containing (A) glycine (100 mmol/l), (B) glycine (100 mmol/l) + glycylglycine (50 mmol/l), and (C) glycylglycine (50 mmol/l) were infused into *proximal* jejunum using the perfusion system; rate of glycine absorption was significantly higher from glycylglycine (C) than from glycine (A). Glycine absorption-rate from solution B was similar to the sum of absorption-rates for glycine from solutions A and C in *every* individual. Luminal disappearance rate of glycylglycine from solutions C and B were similar, rate being significantly faster than total glycine absorption-rate from solution C; this probably indicates 'back-diffusion' of glycine into the lumen following glycylglycine hydrolysis. *Results* confirm therefore that in man, transport mechanisms for glycine and glycylglycine are partly, and possibly wholly, separate.[18]

Effect of glycine and glycylglycine on L-histidine absorption

Using the perfusion system, effects of glycine and glycylglycine on jejunal transfer rate of *L-histidine* were studied in *six* Zambian African men. Data on effect of *L-histidine* on glycylglycine transfer rate was also obtained. Perfusion solutions contained (A) *L-histidine* (100 m-mol 1^{-1}), (B) *L-histidine* (100 m-mol 1^{-1}) + glycylglycine (50 m-mol 1^{-1}), (C) glycylglycine (50 m-mol 1^{-1}), and (D) *Lhistidine* (100 m-mol 1^{-1}) + glycine (100 m-mole 1^{-1}). Whereas presence of glycine significantly impaired absorption-rate of *L-histidine*, glycylglycine had no effect. Presence of *L-histidine* in perfusion fluid did *not* however produce a significant alteration of glycylglycine absorption-rate. When compared with results for glycine absorption-rate in 12 Zambian Africans in another study, presence of *Lhistidine* produced significant impairment of glycine absorption rate. *Results* demonstrate mutual inhibition between *L-histidine* and glycine absorption-rates. Lack of inhibition between *L-histidine* and glycylglycine is consistent with the concept of independent transfer mechanisms for amino-acids and di-peptides in *H sapiens* (*see above*).

Impairment of glycine absorption by glucose and galactose
Competition for absorption between Amino acids and Peptides and Glucose

In animal experiments *in vitro*, interaction *during* absorption between amino-acids and monosaccharides had apparently been assessed. For glucose, nature of mutual interference was unpredictable. In two groups of Zambian Africans mutual inhibition between rates of glucose and galactose (200 mM) and glycine (100 mM) absorption was present. In that study perfusion solutions contained monosaccharide and amino-acid either alone or together, each subject being perfused with three solutions. *Glycine absorption-rate was impaired by approximately 30% by both glucose and galactose*; impairment of monosaccharide absorption-rate by glycine was less. In a further study several concentrations of glucose and glycine were perfused either alone or together. *Glycine absorption-rate from a 20 mM solution was decreased by glucose at concentrations of 200 and 280 mM by approximately 30%.* However, when a solution containing lower concentrations of glycine (10 mM) and glucose (100 mM) was perfused, degree of impairment of glycine absorption-rate was less, and did *not* reach statistical significance; in that study there was also no significant impairment of glucose absorption-rate by low glycine concentration. Similar impairment, but to a lesser degree (19%), of glycine absorption-rate from glycylglycine (50 mM) by glucose (200 mM) was also demonstrated.[19]

Further confirmation that amino-acids (alone or with a monosaccharide) utilise a separate transfer mechanism from glycylglycine.

To investigate competition for intestinal transport between amino-acids and monosaccharides, iso-osmotic solutions containing: (A) 100 m-mol glycine 1^{-1}, (B) 100 m-mole glycine + 200 m-mol monosaccharide (glucose or galactose) 1^{-1}, and (C) 200 m-mol monosaccharide 1^{-1}, were successively perfused into upper jejunum of *12* African Zambian patients, none having *clinical* evidence of either malnutrition or small-intestinal disease. By using the perfusion system, rate of absorption was calculated. *Presence of glucose and galactose produced significant impairment (up to 50%) of glycine absorption-rate.* There was also a significant decrease in uptake of both monosaccharides from solutions in which glycine was present. Should this observation also apply to other amino-acids it could have a significant practical value in those on a high carbohydrate diet with marginal concentration of *essential* amino-acids, and thus have special importance when jejunal mucosa is damaged in *severe* malnutrition or gastrointestinal infection.

Is there mutual interference between L-methionine and glucose during absorption?

Using the perfusion system (*see above*) rates of absorption of *L-methionine* and glucose were assessed in *eight* relatively normal Zambian Africans; effect of each substrate on absorption of the other was also investigated. Solutions contained (A) 100 m-mol 1^{-1} *L methionine*, (B) 100 m-mol 1^{-1} *L-methionine* + 150 m-mol 1^{-1} glucose and (C) 150 m-mol 1^{-1} glucose. Presence of glucose did *not* significantly alter mean absorption-rate of *L-methionine*; in *six* subjects, rate of *L-methionine* absorption from solution B being less than from solution A, but showed an individual difference in effect of glucose on *L-methionine* absorption. Presence of *L-methionine* in perfusing fluid did *not* significantly alter mean absorption-rate of glucose.[20]

Further studies on glucose and glycine absorption:

To investigate effect of luminal concentration on mutual inhibitive glycine and glucose on absorption-rates, *18* convalescent Zambian Africans *without* clinical evidence of intestinal disease or malnutrition underwent constant intrajejunal infusions with these solutes alone or together. The perfusion system was again used, and solutions containing (A) glycine (B) glycine + glucose, and (C) glucose, all rendered iso-osmotic with sodium chloride, were perfused in random order. Concentration of glycine was either 10 or 20 mM, and that of glucose either 100, 200 or 280 mM. By reference to the non-absorbable marker, absorption-rates of solutes and water were calculated. At glucose concentration of 200 or 280 mM, but not 100 mM, *mean rate of glycine absorption was decreased by approximately 30%.* Glucose absorption-rates were *not* significantly altered by presence of glycine. Taken in conjunction with results of a previous investigation, these results are consistent with separate mechanisms for glycine absorption in man, one being inhibited by glucose at high intraluminal concentration.

Using the perfusion technique *in vivo*, absorption-rates of glucose – from glucose (200 mmol l^{-1}) and maltose (100 mmol l^{-1}) solutions – were measured in *six* Zambian African adults. In each, rate of glucose absorption from maltose was greater than that from the glucose solution. Difference between mean rate was approximately 15% and is statistically significant.[21]

Conclusions

I had thus obtained much original data on chemicals which have potential importance in nutrition in Zambia. In addition, I had:

1. established the *lactase* status of the vast majority of adult Zambian Africans,
2. demonstrated an inhibitive effect of *systemic infection* on absorption of several vitally important dietary substances,
3. thrown a 'ray of light' on intestinal absorption mechanisms of dietary components in Zambian Africans, and
4. confirmed that amino-acids present in a staple Zambian diet are frequently swamped by saccharides (such as glucose).

In order to assess the efficacy of the perfusion system used in these studies, an initial investigation was undertaken in collaboration with a consultant surgeon at UTH. A major part of research had focused on the effect of *systemic bacterial infection* – most frequently *bacterial lobar pneumonia* and/or *pulmonary tuberculosis* – on absorption of dietary constituents, remembering that the average Zambian lives on a primarily carbohydrate diet with a marginal amount of protein.

Whereas absorption-rate of glycine – an amino-acid and thus a component of most proteins – was increased in presence of infection, that of the di-peptide, glycylglycine was unaltered, while glucose absorption-rate was severely impaired.

Furthermore, these relationships were confirmed by serum total, ɣ-globulin and IgG concentrations in the absence of *overt* presence of infection. I had also extended these into investigation of other amino-acids and perhaps surprisingly demonstrated that this relationship did *not* apply to *all* amino-acids.. However, presence of glucose in perfusing fluid *impaired* absorption-rate of all amino-acids studied. It seemed that these findings were partly dependent on a transfer mechanism involved but separate from that of the di-peptide glycylglycine!

Therefore, although presence of systemic infection conveys a significant influence upon absorption-rate of protein and carbohydrate, this is complex and possibly varies with different amino-acids.

Overall, what had initially seemed to be a relatively simple matter, proved to be extremely complex, the small-intestine possessing numerous separate and complicated mechanisms, many of which are involved in absorption of amino-acids and monosaccharides.

There were notable critics of this research (*see above*). The topic chosen, although perhaps not of immediate relevance, was undoubtedly potentially important to both Zambia and other emerging African nations. I had thus studied interactions between amino-acids and carbohydrates during absorption from the small-intestine. What could possibly be more relevant to a country dependent on marginal protein intake – such as that acquired from consumption of the staple bedrock – maize (sweetcorn).

My previous research in Africa had largely focused on *hypolactasia*. In Kampala, Uganda I had for example demonstrated for the first time that lactose malabsorption, resulting from *lactase* deficiency in the intestinal brush-border is virtually universal in Bantu-speaking Africans, unlike other tribes on that continent. This has been summarised in *The Milk Enzyme*.

I again stress that most studies involved absorption *rate*; this is a direct reflector of *efficiency* of absorption, *not* assessed in most investigations.

Research funding

Research funding in Zambia was difficult. However, for *clinical* studies I received a modest grant from the Rev W H Woodhouse, at the late Prof R A McCance's instigation without which these studies on amino-acid and carbohydrate absorption and interaction would have been impossible! Much research was *basic* and physiological, but highly relevant to an unsophisticated Zambian population in which nutrition was obviously a major topic.

References and notes

1. Anonymous. State Capture: the ANC and its corrupt leaders have brought South Africa almost to its knees. *Times, Lond* 2022; 6 December: 27; Anonymous. *Times of Zambia:* September 1970.
2. G C Cook. Some factors influencing absorption-rates of the digestive products of protein and carbohydrate from the proximal jejunum of man and their possible nutritional implications. *Gut.* 1974; 15: 239-45.
3. G C Cook, R H Carruthers. Reactions of human small-intestine to an intra luminal tube and its importance in jejunal perfusion studies. *Gut* 1974; 15: 545-8.
4. G C Cook, C R Snook. Site of glucose absorption from the intestine of Zambian African subjects. *Am J clin Nutr* 1974; 27: 91-5.
5. G C Cook. *The Milk Enzyme: adventures with the human lactase polymorphism.* Melrose Books Ltd 2015: 120; G C Cook. The practical significance of lactase deficiency in childhood. *J trop Pediatr* 1967; 13: 85-6. G C Cook. Incidence and clinical features of specific hypolactasia in adult man. *Symposia of the Swedish Nutrition Foundation* IX: 1973.
6. G C Cook. N-G Asp, A Dahlqvist. Activities of brush-border lactase, acid β-galactosidase and hetero β-galactosidase in the jejunum of the Zambian African. *Gastroenterology.* 1973; 64: 405-10; G C Cook, N-G Asp, A Dahlqvist. Lactose absorption kinetics in Zambia African subjects. *Br J Nutr* 1973; 30: 519-27.
7. *See:* Note 5 above.
8. G C Cook. *See:* Note 5 above (*J trop Pediatr.*)
9. G C Cook. Impairment of D-xylose absorption in Zambian patients with systemic bacterial infections. *Am J clin Nutr.* 1972; 25: 490-3.
10. G C Cook. Glucose absorption kinetics in Zambian African patients with and without systemic bacterial infections. *Gut* 1971; 12: 1001-6.
11. G C Cook. Increased glycine absorption-rate associated with acute bacterial infections in man. *Br J Nutr* 1973; 29: 377-86.
12. G C Cook. Effect of systemic infections on glycylglycine absorption-rate from the human jejunum in vivo. *Br J Nutr* 1974; 32: 163-7.
13. G C Cook. Relation between glucose absorption-rate and serum globulin concentration in man. *Nature, Lond* 1973; 241: 284-5.
14. G C Cook. Inverse relation between serum IgG concentration and glucose and xylose absorption in Zambian African adults. *Br med J* 1974; ii: 200-1; G C Cook. Relation between malaria, serum ɣ-globulin concentration and

the D-xylose absorption test. *Trans R Soc trop Med Hyg* 1975; 69: 143-5; G C Cook. Intestinal absorption rate of L-methionine in man and the effect of glucose in the perusing fluid. *J Physiol* 1972; 221: 707-14.
15. G C Cook, J O Morgan, A V Hoffbrand. Impairment of folate absorption by systemic bacterial infections. *Lancet* 1974; ii: 1416-7.
16. G C Cook. Jejunal absorption-rates of glucose, glycine and glycylglycine in Zambian African adults with malnutrition. *Br J Nutr* 1974; 32: 503-13; G C Cook. Impairment of glycine absorption by glucose and galactose in man. *J Physiol* 1971; 217: 61-70.
17. G C Cook. *Op cit. See* note 10 above.
18. G C Cook. Comparison of intestinal absorption rates of glycine and glycylglycine in man and the effect of glucose in the perfusing fluid. *Clin Sci* 1972; 43: 443-53.
19. G C Cook. Independent jejunal mechanisms for glycine and glycylglycine transfer in man in vivo. *Br J Nutr* 1973; 30: 13-19.
20. G C Cook. Effect of glycylglycine and glycine on jejunal absorption-rate of L-histidine in man in vivo. *J Physiol* 1974; 237: 187-94;
21. G C Cook. Effect of intraluminal concentrations on the impairment of glycine absorption by glucose in the human jejunum. *Clin Sci* 1972; 43: 525-34; G C Cook. Comparison of absorption-rates of glucose and maltose in man in vivo. *Clin Sci* 1973; 44: 425-8.

Legends to the figures

Fig 1: Group of newly qualified junior doctors in 2023 – on strike for an increase in pay. P Brookes. ***Times, Lond* 2023; 21 September: 25**

Fig 2: Letter from the foremost expert on fructose metabolism (Professor H A Krebs FRS) during my research spell on sucrose at the Department of Medicine, the *Royal Free Hospital School of Medicine.*

Fig. 3: Telegram offering the Chair of Medicine in the University of Zambia to the author.

Fig 4: Letter from Lord Rosenheim FRCP, FRS to Lusaka in which he expressed his great pleasure at being invited to be external examiner in the first final examination in Medicine at the *University of Zambia.*

Fig 5: Britain was at that time afflicted by numerous strikes for an increase in pay with widespread implications. P Brookes. ***Times, Lond* 2023: 2 September: 23.**

Index

A
Aaronovitch, David 4n, 47, 49n
Abdul Aziz Hospital 34
Alzheimer's 29, 39n
   see also dementia
anatomical dissection 9
antibiotics 1, 2, 4n, 8
   and Strep A 51n
anticoagulants 23
anti-vax movement 9
apartheid 31, 53
appendicitis 9
Athenaeum Club 37
Attlee, Clement 41

B
baby boom 10
Baker, Murray 34
Bamford, Dr Tom 9
Bamji, Nariman 20
Barcroft, Henry 17
Barrett, 'Pasty' 24
Bart's Hospital 12, 17
Best, George 39n
   and see Williams, Roger
Biddulph, John 36
Billing, Barbara 28
Bingham, Lady Jane 20, 23
Bloomsbury Group 13
Blunt, Michael 16
Bowden, Ruth 14, 16
Boxall, Lionel 14
Bridges, Robert 24

British Empire 29
British Medical Association 44, 45, 49n, 51n
British Medical Journal 28, 34
British Society of Gastroenterology 27
Brock, Russell 24
Brookes, Peter 39–40
Bryceson, Tony 35
Bull, Sir Graham 34
Burkitt, Denis 54

C
Cameron, David 45
cardiology 23
Carruthers, Richard 56
Carter, Dr 8, 9
Charing Cross Hospital 12
cholera 12, 18n
Chronic Fatigue Syndrome 16
Clinical Science 29
clinical tropical medicine 27, 39n
Clunies-Ross, Dr 9
Compston, Nigel 23
Cook, Professor G C *The Milk Enzyme* 29, 34, 39n, 54, 58, 73, 74n
Cope, James 20
Coram, Thomas 14n
corticosteroids 28, 29
Countess of Lucan
   see Bingham, Lady Jane
Covid-19 5, 6, 37, 43, 46, 47
Crowcroft, Andrew 14

D
Dawson, Tony 28, 54, 56
Day, Brian 14
Day, Michael 14
dementia 29, 39n
    see also Alzheimer's
Dickens, Charles 13, 14n
Dilnot, Sir Andrew 45
diphtheria 45, 46, 51n
Dow, James 27, 28
Down's Syndrome
    see Mongolism
Duckworth, Marjorie ('Daisy') 16

F
Fleming, Alexander 2
Foster-Carter, Dr Aylmer 24
fructose 29
    see also sucrose
Fursden, Paul 14, 15

G
Gardner, Dame Frances 19, 20, 23, 28, 29
gastroenterology 27, 74n
gastrointestinal disease 62, 63, 65
Gibson, John R M 14
Gilchrist, Edith 20
Giles, Peter 15
glaucoma
    see *Hirudo medicinalis*
Greene, Raymond 24
Gunn, 'Willy' 20
Gut 56, 74n
Guy's Hospital 2, 12, 13, 17

H
Hall, Joe 19
Hamilton-Fairley, Sir Neil 35n
Hampstead General Hospital 12, 23
Händel, Georg Friedrich 14n
Harvey, William 53
Heitmueller, Dr Axel 47
hepatitis 29
hepatotoxins 28
Herbert, Mervyn 8, 11n

Hicklin, Tony 16
Hippocrates 12–13
Hirudo medicinalis 24
    see also glaucoma
HM Queen Elizabeth II 54
Hogarth, William 14n
Hospital for Tropical Diseases 35, 36, 37, 42
house appointments 23
Hynes, Martin 24
hypolactasia
    see lactase

I
immunisation 9, 13

J
Jenkins, 'Taffy' 20
Jex-Blake, Sophia 15
Johnson, 'Teddy' 34
Johnson, Boris 2, 5
    and private health care 44
    and social care 45
    and the Covid-19 pandemic 47
    fall of 50n
    how not to be a prime minister 50n

K
Kaunda, Kenneth 53
Keats, John 17
    Keats: a brief life in nine poems and one epitaph (L Miller) 18n
Kempster, Clive (Ronald) 15
Killick, Esther Margaret 16
King's College School 15
Krebs, Professor H A 30
Kursner, Frederick 16

L
lactase 29, 31, 34, 39n, 54, 58, 59, 60–61, 72–73, 74n
    and hypolactasia 29, 56, 58, 59, 60, 61, 73, 74n
    lactase deficiency 73
    lactose malabsorption 73

Lancet 28, 29, 37, 39n, 51n, 75n
Ledingham, Una 20
Lequesne, Leslie 24
lesbianism 14
Levy, Jonathan 28
Lewis, A A G 17
Liebster, Leila 15
Linacre, Thomas 13
    see also Royal College of Physicians
Lions Club 55
Lloyd-Williams, Katharine 13
London Metropolitan archive 20
London School of Hygiene and Tropical Medicine 31, 35, 37, 42
London School of Medicine for Women 2, 13, 14
London Times, The
    A&E delays in v
Lucas-Keene, Mary 16
Lusaka Central Hospital 54

M

Makerere University College 28, 54, 55
malaria 27, 35n, 46, 62, 63, 74n
    Melfloquine 35
malnutrition 55, 56, 59, 61, 62, 64, 65, 66, 67, 68, 70, 75n
    and heart attacks 55
    childhood malnutrition (marasmus) 59
Manson, Sir Patrick 27, 35, 35n
Manson-Bahr, Clinton 35
    Manson's Tropical Diseases 35
Marburg disease 46
Marsden, William 12, 13
    Surgeon Compassionate: the story of Dr William Marsden (F Sandwith) 18n
McCance, Prof R A 73
McDowell, R J S 17
McIntyre, Neil 28
McLeod, Cameron 23
Medical Research Council 34, 54
Medical Research Council's Child Nutrition Unit 29

medicine
    and world population 10
Middlesex Hospital 12, 17, 24
Minton, Joseph 23, 24
mitral stenosis 20
Mongolism (Down's Syndrome) 9
monkeypox 46
Monroe, Dowling 14
Moore, Roland 16
Moran, Maureen 3
Mulago Hospital 28, 54
Murley, Sir Reginald 24
myocardial infarction 23, 46

N

National Health Service (NHS)
    ambulance delays 44
    and Brexit 48
    and care system staff turnover
    and Covid-19 43
    and social care 43
    cradle-to-grave healthcare 6
    current popular opinion of 5
    deterioration of healthcare service 42, 42–43, 47, 48
    excessive running costs of 6
    financial governance of 5
    free at the point of service 5
    inception of 1
    medicine before NHS era 8, 42
    political management of 6, 43–44
    state of today 2–3
    strikes in 44
National Service 25, 27, 39n
Nelson, George 54
NHS Act 15, 41
NHS vacancies 41
Nicholson, Howard 24

P

Paget's Disease of Bone 9
Paneth, Matthew 24
Papworth, Maurice 28
penicillin 2
Peters, Michael 24

pneumonia 9, 62, 72
poliomyelitis 9, 45, 46
    Salk and Sabin 45, 49n
Price-Thomas, Clement 24
Princess Alice Hospital 23

Q
Quarterly Journal of Medicine 29
Queen Victoria Royal Charter 12
Qvist, George 15n, 19, 20

R
Ramsay, Melvyn 20, 51n
    and Royal Free disease 20
rat-bite fever 46
rheumatic fever 20
    see also mitral stenosis
Richardson, Peter 16
Robert, Paul 16
Roberts, David 14
Robson, Sir Kenneth 24, 27
Rosenheim, Max 31, 33
Rosser, Reg 15
Royal Brompton Hospital 24, 27
Royal College of Physicians of London 13, 24, 31, 33
Royal Free Disease
    see also Chronic Fatigue Syndrome
    see also Ramsay, Melvyn
Royal Free Hospital 12, 13, 16, 19, 20, 23, 28, 51n, 54
    An Illustrated History of the Royal Free Hospital (L A Amidon) 18n
Royal Free Hospital School of Medicine viii, 12, 13, 14, 30
Royal Nigerian Army 25
Royal Northern Hospital 24
Ryman, Brenda 16

S
'Shy-bladder Syndrome' (paruresis) 15n
Salmond, Margaret 16
scarlet fever 9
schistosomiasis 27
Sherlock, Dame Sheila 28, 29, 53
Smith, Dr C E Gordon 35, 37
social care 45
    see also National Health Service
Society of Apothecaries 14
St Bartholomew's Hospital 13, 54, 56
St George's Hospital 27, 28
St Mary's Hospital Medical School 16, 23
St Olave's Hospital 16
St Thomas's Hospital 13, 17
sucrose 29–30, 34, 46, 76
    see also fructose
Suga, Yoshihide 10
Sunak, Rishi 48
Sunday Times 1, 4n, 7n, 18n, 22n, 41, 49n, 50n, 51n, 52n
    doctors' pay 51n
    GP charges 52n
    Lord Lucan mystery 22n
    maternity care crisis 50n
    NHS and political leadership 49n, 50n
    NHS strikes 50n, 51n
    NHS vacancies 49n
    problems in NHS 41n
    Strep A medicine prices 51n
    students and medical schools 18n
    working hours crisis 1, 4n, 7n, 49n
Sylvester, Rachel 43, 51n
syphilis 13

T
Tembo, James 54
Thatcher, Margaret 2
The Times of Zambia 54
Third World
    medicine in 1
Thucydides 13
Toxocara canis 35n
tropical medicine 27, 34, 35, 36, 37
Tropical Medicine Research Board 54
Trump, Donald 44
tuberculosis 9, 13, 24, 27, 36, 46, 62, 72

U

Underwood, Mary 16, 17
University College Hospital 54
University College, London 24, 37
University of London 20, 34
University of Zambia 33, 55

V

Victorian remedies 8
vitamin D 29, 39n, 59

W

Walker, Geoffrey 28
Welby, Justin (105th Archbishop of Canterbury) 29
Wellcome Chair 35n
Westminster Hospital 14
Williams, Dr Cecily 64
Williams, Roger 28, 39n
    and George Best 39n
Woodhouse, Rev W H 73
Wood, Paul 24
women in medicine 2
    The Charge of the Parasols: women's entry to the Medical Profession (C Blake) 18n
Woodruff, Alan 27, 31, 35, 35n, 36, 37, 42
Woolf, Virginia 13
Wright, Sampson 17
Wakefield, Andrew 13, 18n
    and aetiology of Crohn's Disease 13
    The Doctor who fooled the world: Andrew Wakefield's war on vaccines (B Deer) 18n
Williams, Emlyn 23, 24